Teenage Pregnancy

Opposing Viewpoints ®

Other Books of Related Interest

OPPOSING VIEWPOINTS SERIES

Abortion
Adoption
American Values
America's Youth
The Family
Teens at Risk

CURRENT CONTROVERSIES SERIES

The Abortion Controversy
Teen Pregnancy and Parenting

AT ISSUE SERIES

The Ethics of Abortion
Sex Education
Single-Parent Families
Teen Sex

Teenage Pregnancy

Opposing Viewpoints ®

Auriana Ojeda, *Book Editor*

Daniel Leone, *President*
Bonnie Szumski, *Publisher*
Scott Barbour, *Managing Editor*

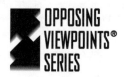

OPPOSING
VIEWPOINTS®
SERIES

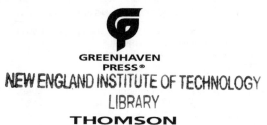

GREENHAVEN
PRESS®

THOMSON
————————— ™
GALE

San Diego • Detroit • New York • San Francisco • Cleveland
New Haven, Conn. • Waterville, Maine • London • Munich

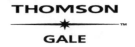

THOMSON

GALE

LIBRARY OF CONGRESS CATALOGING-IN-PUBLICATION DATA
Teenage pregnancy : opposing viewpoints / Auriana Ojeda, book editor.
    p. cm. — (Opposing viewpoints series)
Includes bibliographical references and index.
ISBN 0-7377-1243-0 (pbk. : alk. paper) —
ISBN 0-7377-1244-9 (lib. bdg. : alk. paper)
    1. Teenage mothers. 2. Teenage pregnancy. 3. Teenage fathers. I. Ojeda, Auriana, 1977– . II. Opposing viewpoints series (Unnumbered)
HQ759.4 .T46 2003
306.874'3—dc21   2002023543

Printed in the United States of America

"Congress shall make
no law...abridging the
freedom of speech, or of
the press."

First Amendment to the U.S. Constitution

The basic foundation of our democracy is the First
Amendment guarantee of freedom of expression.
The Opposing Viewpoints Series is dedicated to the
concept of this basic freedom and the idea that it is
more important to practice it than to enshrine it.

Contents

Why Consider Opposing Viewpoints?   9

Introduction   12

Chapter 1: Is Teenage Pregnancy a Serious Problem?

Chapter Preface   17

1. Teenage Pregnancy Is a Serious Problem   19
   Kristin A. Moore and Barbara W. Sugland

2. The Media Exaggerate the Problem of Teenage
   Pregnancy   27
   Janine Jackson

3. Teenagers Can Make Good Parents   33
   Jasmine Miller

4. Teenage Parents Face Daunting Challenges   42
   Lisa W.

Periodical Bibliography   46

Chapter 2: What Factors Contribute to Teenage Pregnancy?

Chapter Preface   48

1. Older Men Contribute to Teenage Pregnancy   49
   Part I: *Linda Valdez;* Part II: *Ellen Goodman*

2. Older Men May Not Contribute to Teenage
   Pregnancy   54
   Laura Duberstein Lindberg et al.

3. Sexual Abuse Contributes to Teenage Pregnancy   63
   Jacqueline L. Stock et al.

4. Poor Life Circumstances Contribute to Teenage
   Pregnancy   71
   Richard T. Cooper

5. A Lack of Accurate Sex Information Contributes to
   Teenage Pregnancy   78
   Jo Ann Wentzel

Periodical Bibliography   83

**Chapter 3: What Options Are Available to
 Pregnant Teenagers?**

Chapter Preface   85

1. Abortion Is an Option for Pregnant Teenagers   86
   Elisabeth Pruden

2. Abortion Should Not Be an Option for Pregnant
   Teenagers   93
   Liz Kleemeier

3. Adoption Is an Option for Pregnant Teenagers   98
   Rebecca Lanning

4. Adoption May Not Be an Option for Pregnant
   Teenagers   106
   Katha Pollitt

Periodical Bibliography   110

**Chapter 4: How Can Teenage Pregnancy Be
 Reduced?**

Chapter Preface   112

1. Abstinence-Only Sex Education Can Reduce
   Teenage Pregnancy   113
   Lakita Garth

2. Abstinence-Only Sex Education Cannot Reduce
   Teenage Pregnancy   123
   National Abortion and Reproductive Rights Action League

3. Traditional Sex Education Can Reduce Teenage
   Pregnancy   134
   Planned Parenthood Federation of America

4. Welfare Reform May Reduce Teenage Pregnancy   143
   Isabel V. Sawhill

5. Welfare Benefits Do Not Reduce Teenage
   Pregnancy   154
   Kathleen Sylvester

6. Male Involvement Programs Can Reduce Teenage
   Pregnancy   164
   Kristin A. Moore, Anne K. Driscoll, and Theodora Ooms

Periodical Bibliography   176

For Further Discussion   177
Organizations to Contact   180
Bibliography of Books   186
Index   188

Why Consider Opposing Viewpoints?

"The only way in which a human being can make some approach to knowing the whole of a subject is by hearing what can be said about it by persons of every variety of opinion and studying all modes in which it can be looked at by every character of mind. No wise man ever acquired his wisdom in any mode but this."

John Stuart Mill

In our media-intensive culture it is not difficult to find differing opinions. Thousands of newspapers and magazines and dozens of radio and television talk shows resound with differing points of view. The difficulty lies in deciding which opinion to agree with and which "experts" seem the most credible. The more inundated we become with differing opinions and claims, the more essential it is to hone critical reading and thinking skills to evaluate these ideas. Opposing Viewpoints books address this problem directly by presenting stimulating debates that can be used to enhance and teach these skills. The varied opinions contained in each book examine many different aspects of a single issue. While examining these conveniently edited opposing views, readers can develop critical thinking skills such as the ability to compare and contrast authors' credibility, facts, argumentation styles, use of persuasive techniques, and other stylistic tools. In short, the Opposing Viewpoints Series is an ideal way to attain the higher-level thinking and reading skills so essential in a culture of diverse and contradictory opinions.

In addition to providing a tool for critical thinking, Opposing Viewpoints books challenge readers to question their own strongly held opinions and assumptions. Most people form their opinions on the basis of upbringing, peer pressure, and personal, cultural, or professional bias. By reading carefully balanced opposing views, readers must directly confront new ideas as well as the opinions of those with whom they disagree. This is not to simplistically argue that everyone who reads opposing views will—or should—change his or her opinion. Instead, the series enhances readers' understanding of their own views by encouraging confrontation with opposing ideas. Careful examination of others' views can lead to the readers' understanding of the logical inconsistencies in their own opinions, perspective on why they hold an opinion, and the consideration of the possibility that their opinion requires further evaluation.

Evaluating Other Opinions

To ensure that this type of examination occurs, Opposing Viewpoints books present all types of opinions. Prominent spokespeople on different sides of each issue as well as well-known professionals from many disciplines challenge the reader. An additional goal of the series is to provide a forum for other, less known, or even unpopular viewpoints. The opinion of an ordinary person who has had to make the decision to cut off life support from a terminally ill relative, for example, may be just as valuable and provide just as much insight as a medical ethicist's professional opinion. The editors have two additional purposes in including these less known views. One, the editors encourage readers to respect others' opinions—even when not enhanced by professional credibility. It is only by reading or listening to and objectively evaluating others' ideas that one can determine whether they are worthy of consideration. Two, the inclusion of such viewpoints encourages the important critical thinking skill of objectively evaluating an author's credentials and bias. This evaluation will illuminate an author's reasons for taking a particular stance on an issue and will aid in readers' evaluation of the author's ideas.

It is our hope that these books will give readers a deeper understanding of the issues debated and an appreciation of the complexity of even seemingly simple issues when good and honest people disagree. This awareness is particularly important in a democratic society such as ours in which people enter into public debate to determine the common good. Those with whom one disagrees should not be regarded as enemies but rather as people whose views deserve careful examination and may shed light on one's own.

Thomas Jefferson once said that "difference of opinion leads to inquiry, and inquiry to truth." Jefferson, a broadly educated man, argued that "if a nation expects to be ignorant and free . . . it expects what never was and never will be." As individuals and as a nation, it is imperative that we consider the opinions of others and examine them with skill and discernment. The Opposing Viewpoints Series is intended to help readers achieve this goal.

David L. Bender and Bruno Leone,
Founders

Greenhaven Press anthologies primarily consist of previously published material taken from a variety of sources, including periodicals, books, scholarly journals, newspapers, government documents, and position papers from private and public organizations. These original sources are often edited for length and to ensure their accessibility for a young adult audience. The anthology editors also change the original titles of these works in order to clearly present the main thesis of each viewpoint and to explicitly indicate the opinion presented in the viewpoint. These alterations are made in consideration of both the reading and comprehension levels of a young adult audience. Every effort is made to ensure that Greenhaven Press accurately reflects the original intent of the authors included in this anthology.

Introduction

"Early out-of-wedlock childbearing greatly compounds the problem [of poverty]."

—Isabel V. Sawhill

"Existing poverty, alcohol and drug abuse, disrupted families, and violence are the breeding ground for young people who are at greater risk for early sexual activity and too-early parenting."

—Sheila Beachum-Bilby

According to the Alan Guttmacher Institute (AGI), a nonprofit agency that focuses on sexual and reproductive health research, policy analysis, and public education, teenage pregnancy has adverse consequences for the parents, the child, and society. Pregnant teens are less likely to complete high school and attend college than teenagers who avoid pregnancy. Many teenage parents live below the poverty level and rely on welfare. The children of teenage parents receive inadequate medical care, have more problems in school, and spend more time in prison than children of adult parents. The National Campaign to Prevent Teen Pregnancy (NCPTP) claims that teenage childbearing costs society about $6.9 billion annually; this estimate includes welfare and food stamp benefits, medical care expenses, lost tax revenue (teenage childbearing affects the parents' work patterns), incarceration expenses, and foster care. In an effort to reduce teenage pregnancy and the problems associated with it, policymakers have recently focused on what causes the widespread poverty and welfare dependence that teen moms experience and have attempted to devise solutions to these problems.

Some social critics argue that because pregnancy limits a teenager's opportunities for education and well-paying jobs, many are forced to accept welfare to support themselves and their children. Only 64 percent of teen moms graduate from high school or earn a general education diploma within two years after they would have graduated compared with 94 percent of teenage girls who do not give birth. This lack of education increases the risk of poverty and welfare dependence by severely restricting a young parent's opportunity for a lucrative job and financial independence. According to Kids Count, a project by the Annie E. Casey Foundation, "The failure to go further in school can limit the mother's employment options and increase the likelihood that she and her family will be poor. And the roughly one-fifth of adolescent moms who have more than one child are even more economically vulnerable. They might further delay finishing high school, putting them at greater risk of being slotted into low-wage jobs or facing prolonged unemployment, poverty, and welfare." According to Child Trends, a nonprofit research organization, nearly 80 percent of teen moms eventually go on welfare, and 55 percent of all mothers on welfare were teenagers at the time their first child was born.

The absence of many teenage fathers further increases a young mother's risk of poverty and welfare dependence. The teenage marriage rate has declined in recent decades, leaving many young mothers without a husband's financial support. Although the teenage pregnancy rate in the 1950s and 1960s was higher than today, the teenage marriage rate was also higher; in 1960 the percentage of unmarried teenage births was 15 percent, compared with 75 percent today. Many social commentators argue that the decline in teenage marriage has contributed to the rise in poverty and welfare dependence of single mothers. According to scholar Patrick F. Fagan, "The major change in teen pregnancy is not the numbers or rates of teen pregnancy, but the massive abandonment of marriage. . . . Having a baby out of wedlock is the major way to derail progress towards a future stable family life with its attendant more comfortable domestic economy." Fagan and others maintain that without the bonds of marriage to hold couples together, many young fathers abandon young mothers and their children to poverty and welfare dependence.

Other social critics argue that poverty and adverse life circumstances foster teenage pregnancy, rather than result from it. Data from the American Academy of Pediatrics reveal that about 83 percent of adolescents who give birth and

13

61 percent who have abortions come from poor or low-income families. According to professor Michael A. Carrera,

> Unfortunately, many teen males and females do not have the good fortune of living in [stable family] situations and do not see much of a future for themselves. Most young people see little employment opportunity around them and will probably face a life of low economic status, ever-present racism, and inadequate opportunities for quality education. . . . Under such conditions, it is no wonder that some young people, instead of becoming industrious and hopeful, become sexually intimate for a short-term sense of comfort, and ultimately become profoundly fatalistic.

These teenagers perceive few opportunities to achieve better circumstances than they were raised in; therefore, they are less inspired to avoid pregnancy and childbearing than teens from more affluent backgrounds.

As a possible solution to the social and economic costs of welfare-dependent teenage mothers, in 1996 Congress passed the "Personal Responsibility and Work Opportunity Reconciliation Act," otherwise known as the welfare reform bill. One intention of the bill was to reduce the number of teenage and out-of-wedlock pregnancies by making benefits more difficult for teenage parents to obtain. The law forbids states from using federal funds to provide assistance to unmarried parents under the age of eighteen who have a child that is at least twelve weeks old unless the parents have completed high school or are enrolled in school or training programs. In addition, in order to receive benefits, teenage parents under the age of eighteen must live with a parent or in another adult-supervised setting, which states may assist teenage parents in locating. States are also given the power to deny welfare benefits to unmarried teenage parents under the age of eighteen. Supporters of welfare reform hope that these provisions, along with pregnancy prevention education programs, can decrease the number of teenage pregnancies and reduce the resulting burden on taxpayers.

Critics of the welfare bill argue that many of its provisions will result in increased poverty among young mothers and children who rely on welfare as their primary source of income. According to the AGI, most of the provisions "rely on disincentives—the threat of punitive measures down the line—to discourage teenage childbearing." This strategy assumes that young women intentionally get pregnant in order to receive welfare checks. However, statistics from the AGI suggest that 85 percent of teenage pregnancies are unintentional. The AGI concludes that these components of welfare reform

> are targeted largely at the very small proportion of young women who are likely to go on public assistance immediately upon the birth of their baby. Yet, very often there is a lag—sometimes of several years—between the time most teenagers who eventually become welfare-dependent give birth and when they actually begin to receive [welfare] benefits. These women, presumably, are not expecting to go on welfare when they have a child and therefore are unlikely to change their behavior as a result of restrictions on welfare eligibility related to childbearing.

The AGI and others maintain that addressing the causes of teenage pregnancy, such as poverty and unfavorable life circumstances, will more effectively reduce the rate of teenage parenting and its accompanying problems.

Supporters of the 1996 welfare reform bill hope that it can defray some of the social costs of teenage pregnancy. Others maintain that society will benefit most from solving the social and economic factors that contribute to teenage pregnancy. *Teenage Pregnancy: Opposing Viewpoints* presents these and other issues in the following chapters: Is Teenage Pregnancy a Serious Problem? What Factors Contribute to Teenage Pregnancy? What Options Are Available to Pregnant Teenagers? How Can Teenage Pregnancy Be Reduced? Examination of these arguments should give readers a thorough understanding of the problems surrounding teenage pregnancy.

CHAPTER 1

Is Teenage Pregnancy a Serious Problem?

Chapter Preface

The 1950s and 1960s saw the highest recorded rates of teenage childbearing in the United States, as 90 out of 1,000 teenage girls gave birth in the late 1950s. Statistics reflect a significant decline to 48.7 births per 1,000 teenagers in 1999. Despite this decrease, many people argue that the problems associated with teenage pregnancy and childbearing are more serious today than they were in the 1950s and 1960s.

Some people contend that the problem lies not in the rates of pregnancy and childbearing, but in the decline of marriage among teenagers. In 1960, the percentage of unmarried teenage births was 15 percent, but today about 80 percent of teenage pregnancies and 75 percent of teenage births are to unmarried girls. In the 1950s and 1960s, premarital sex was widely considered immoral, and the lack of reliable birth control often quickly revealed a teenager's indiscretion. The desire to avoid the social stigma that accompanied an unwed pregnancy forced many teenagers into shotgun weddings. While these marriages may not have been ideal, divorce was rare and young mothers had the financial security of husbands and help raising their children.

The 1960s and 1970s brought the sexual revolution, birth control, and the legalization of abortion in 1973. Many experts argue that these social changes shifted the public view of sexuality and marriage. The freedom that accompanied personal control over one's fertility manifested as freer sexual behavior and independence. Many women were acquiring more education and entering the workforce, and they no longer needed the security of marriage and a husband. Although unwanted pregnancies still occurred, many women found single-motherhood a more attractive option than marriage.

While the late 1960s and 1970s heightened the independence of many women and girls, the decline of the two-parent family created problems that the 1950s and early 1960s had avoided. Today, experts estimate that the social cost of teenage pregnancy and childbearing, including lost tax revenues, public assistance, child health care, foster care, and the criminal justice system, totals about $7 billion annually. Nearly 80 percent of teenage mothers eventually go on welfare. Many people argue that although teenage marriages that resulted from pregnancy in the 1950s and early 1960s were not perfect, they created fewer costs to society and provided children with the best chances for success. As stated by scholar Patrick F. Fagan, "There is virtual unanimity among researchers that family structure has a massive impact on income, and that children who grow up in intact married families have the best chance of empowerment, of economic independence in their adulthood."

While teenage pregnancy was considered a moral issue in the 1950s and early 1960s, society today views it as an irresponsible act that may result in an increased burden on taxpayers. The viewpoints in the following chapter address how serious the problem of teenage pregnancy is for society.

> "The U.S. teenage birth rate remains two
> to ten times higher than teenage birth
> rates in other industrialized nations."

Teenage Pregnancy Is a Serious Problem

Kristin A. Moore and Barbara W. Sugland

In the following viewpoint, Kristin A. Moore and Barbara W. Sugland contend that teenage pregnancy is a serious problem because teenage parents complete fewer years of school than older parents, and this lack of education undermines their employment prospects. In addition, the children of teenage parents often do poorly in school and suffer behavioral problems. Moore and Sugland argue that community efforts, such as educational programs, are necessary to combat the problem of adolescent pregnancy. Kristin A. Moore is the president of Child Trends, a nonprofit, nonpartisan research organization dedicated to studying children, youth, and families; Barbara W. Sugland is a senior research associate at Child Trends.

As you read, consider the following questions:

1. What problems do the authors associate with living in a single-parent family?
2. What are three risk factors for teenage pregnancy, as described by the authors?
3. As cited by the authors, what are three factors that adolescents suggest might reduce teenage pregnancy?

Recent declines in the teenage birth rate are encouraging, but we see little cause for complacency. The U.S. teenage birth rate remains two to ten times higher than teenage birth rates in other industrialized nations. Teenage parents complete fewer years of school than older parents, and their limited educational attainment undermines their employment prospects. Their children are at greater risk of poor birth outcomes and, as they grow older, have poorer cognitive, behavioral, and school outcomes. Finally, because the vast majority of teenage births (76 percent) occur outside of marriage, many teenage mothers and their children face the challenges associated with living in a single-parent family, including lower income and greater demands on a mother's time and attention.

Researchers at Child Trends, a nonprofit, nonpartisan research center, have studied this issue for two decades from several vantage points. We track and analyze trends in teenage sexual behavior, pregnancy, and childbearing. We study the antecedents and consequences of teenage childbearing. We explore factors that might discourage too-early parenthood, as well as those that place adolescents at risk. We examine the effectiveness of programs and cultural messages intended to discourage teenage child-bearing, and we empirically test hypotheses to explain changes in the teenage birth rate nationally and variation in teenage birth rates across the states.

As a result, we are continually adding to our understanding of what contributes to teenage childbearing and what might discourage it. While the puzzle is incomplete, enough pieces are in place to offer a better understanding of this complex issue.

Recent Trends in Teenage Childbearing

Teenage birth rates have decreased in the United States for six consecutive years (1992–1997, the most recent years for which data are available). This sustained downward trend was a welcome departure from the previous five-year period (1986–1991), during which rates rose by 24 percent. These increases in the late 1980s were particularly troubling because they followed more than 25 years of declining teenage birth rates in the United States. In 1997, the teenage birth rate was 52.9 births per 1,000 females ages 15– 19. This rate represents a significant (15 percent) decrease since 1991. Nevertheless, the 1997 teenage birth rate is still higher than the 1986 rate of 50.2, the nation's lowest in more than half a century.

The decline in the teenage birth rate has occurred in every state, suggesting that the decrease in the national rate reflects broad, society-wide changes rather than changes limited to one part of the country or to one group of teenagers. Still, teenage birth rates vary widely across the states. Several states, including Vermont, New Hampshire, Minnesota, North Dakota, Massachusetts, and Maine, have teenage birth rates at or around 32 births per 1,000 females ages 15–19. In contrast, several other states, including Mississippi, Arizona, Texas, and Arkansas, have teenage birth rates at or above 74 births per 1,000 females ages 15–19. Identifying the multiple factors that account for this great variation across states is no easy task, but is a question that researchers are actively pursuing at Child Trends and elsewhere.

White teenagers have consistently had lower birth rates than African American or Hispanic teenagers, although the gap between whites and nonwhites is getting smaller. While birth rates have fallen for both white and African American teenagers in recent years, the decline has been more pronounced for African Americans. The teenage birth rate for African Americans fell by 22 percent between 1991 and 1997, from 116 to 90 births per 1,000 females ages 15–19. In contrast, birth rates among white teenagers declined by 16 percent over the same time period, from 43 to 36 births per 1,000 females ages 15–19.

Trends among Hispanic teenagers are less promising. Between 1991 and 1995, there was virtually no change in the Hispanic teenage birth rate, so that by 1995, Hispanics had a higher teenage birth rate (107) than either African Americans or whites. The Hispanic teenage birth rate decreased notably in 1996 and 1997, however, declining to 99 births per 1,000 females ages 15–19 in 1997. . . .

Much remains to be done in the cultural, political, and programmatic arenas to continue and accelerate the current decrease in teenage childbearing. The volatility of the teenage birth rate over the last few decades—down significantly in the 1960s and 1970s, up substantially in the late 1980s and early 1990s, and now heading down again—reminds us that the tide could turn yet again. Moreover, the number of teenagers is increasing rapidly, threatening to increase the number of teenage births if further substantial reductions in the rate of childbearing do not occur.

So what is likely to bring about further reductions in teenage childbearing? At Child Trends, we approach this question from several perspectives, including review of the basic research literature and of rigorous evaluations of programs intended to discourage teenage childbearing; qualitative research involving focus groups with adolescents; and analyses of existing and new data. From these varied perspectives, we offer the following thoughts.

Who Is at Risk of a Teenage Birth?

A review of the basic research literature helps us identify those children and adolescents at heightened risk of teenage parenthood. Armed with this information, policymakers and service providers can test interventions that might lower this risk. Research consistently highlights the following factors that place children and youth at risk of teenage childbearing:

• *Family problems.* Teenagers are at higher risk of early pregnancy and parenting if their families provide too little monitoring, are characterized by poor communication between parents and children, fail to teach values or encourage goal-setting, and do little to counteract damaging cultural and media messages. Families also need to protect children from coercive sex. States, communities, and private organizations should explore programs to strengthen families or provide teenagers with extra social and emotional support to lessen the risk of teenage parenthood.

• *School problems.* Teenagers who are below their expected grade levels, whose school achievement is low, and who have dropped out are two to five times more likely to have a child by the time they would have completed high school. This factor suggests that programs to enhance school performance and engagement in learning as early as preschool and the elementary grades are a promising approach to reduce teenage childbearing. As we discuss later in this article, new research by Child Trends lends further support to this hypothesis.

• *Behavior problems.* Teenagers and younger children with behavior problems in school, who smoke, drink, or use drugs, and who engage in delinquent behavior are more likely to become teenage parents. Thus, interventions that address problem behaviors among children in general may also reduce childbearing among troubled youth. Again, states might initiate efforts to improve behavior well before the teenage years.

• *Poverty and low income.* Many children and adolescents who grow up poor (especially those who grow up in extremely poor communities), see little likelihood that they will escape poverty in adulthood. When youth perceive limited opportunities for themselves, they are often less motivated to avoid pregnancy, and early childbearing. On the other hand, better employment opportunities are associated with a lower probability of a teenage birth. Activities that enhance adolescents' economic opportunities and present them with positive options for the future may therefore increase their motivation to avoid pregnancy.

What Are We Doing Right?

For at least two decades, communities, schools, and service providers have tried a range of approaches to prevent teenage childbearing. To date, few have convincingly demonstrated "large, sustained, and clearly documented" successes [as stated by K.A. Moore and B.W. Sugland]. Most are small, short-term projects. Many are not sufficiently grounded in research on child and adolescent development, and most do not have a strong evaluation component.

Abstinence programs, for example, have become increasingly popular in states and communities across the country. To date, however, none has been rigorously evaluated so it is impossible to say with certainty whether they are effective in bringing about large declines in teenage pregnancy. Temporary Assistance for Needy Families (TANF) funding for abstinence programs offers a good opportunity to put rigorous evaluations in place.

Many traditional sex education programs in the public

schools, which generally provide factual information to high school students, have been rigorously evaluated. Although such programs increase knowledge, many of these programs have not demonstrated great success at changing behavior. For example, they appear to have little effect on whether teenagers initiate sex or use contraception. School-based clinics providing adolescent health services (but not always providing contraception) have also not shown convincing evidence of reducing teenage pregnancies or births.

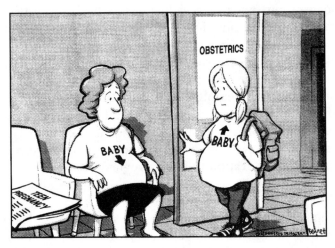

Bennett. © by Clay Bennett. Reprinted by permission of United Media Enterprises.

On the other hand, sex education that combines information with skill-building activities (such as developing specific negotiation and refusal skills) appears more promising. These kinds of programs have resulted in short delays in the initiation of sexual intercourse among some groups and have proven moderately effective at improving contraceptive use among teenagers.

In the long run, programs that focus on improving educational and employment outcomes—but not explicitly on preventing teenage childbearing—may be a good bet. . . . New research from Child Trends suggests that programs and approaches that emphasize keeping girls in school and engaged in learning may also lessen the incidence of teenage child-bearing.

What Do the Kids Say?

To augment and check conclusions based on research, Child Trends has conducted focus groups with white, black, and Hispanic youth in several cities, asking them to identify those factors that are most likely to motivate them to avoid pregnancy. In many cases, their answers were consistent with the research and program evaluations summarized above. In other cases, they suggest intriguing new directions for research and programs.

The factors that adolescents suggested would increase their motivation to avoid pregnancy included:

• Encourage adolescents to set goals for themselves, help them understand the steps necessary to reach those goals, and how certain actions and behaviors make those goals harder to attain.

• Support and strengthen families by helping parents and adolescents communicate effectively about sexuality, peer relationships, school, and the future, and by increasing family involvement and support in all aspects of teenagers' lives.

• Provide a broader form of sexuality education that includes building the skills and confidence to handle friendships and romantic relationships, as well as providing information on the variety of available contraceptive methods, how to use them, and how to obtain them.

• Make affordable, confidential contraceptive services available to teenagers.

• Address larger societal influences that undercut messages about responsible sexual behavior and the value of planning for the future. These include the need for more positive adult role models, pervasive messages in the media that sex has few consequences, and easy access to drugs and alcohol.

Information from additional focus groups also indicates that how teenagers perceive their educational, social, and career opportunities affects how motivated they are to avoid early childbearing. This is consistent with data analyses that suggest that adolescents' future opportunities affect the likelihood of a teenage birth. But our work also indicates that the pathway from perceptions of economic opportunity to avoiding a teenage birth is not direct. Instead, perceptions of opportunity influence how adolescents view other activities that protect against childbearing, such as school-related academic, extracurricular, and social activities. If future quantitative research examining the link between perceptions, school engagement, and teenage childbearing supports this finding, then this research has implications beyond avoiding teenage pregnancy and may offer insights into helping teenagers avoid a host of negative behaviors.

Public discussions of how to prevent teenage pregnancy have become increasingly sophisticated. To a large extent, policymakers, service providers, and the public recognize the complexity of the issues surrounding teenage childbearing and are less likely to seek or accept quick and easy answers. While the puzzle is not complete, one part of it is increasingly clear: different approaches are likely to be effective with different adolescents. For many, delaying sex will be an effective strategy. For others, information, skill-building, and access to contraceptive services will help. And for all youth, long-term strategies that address the antecedents of teenage childbearing—family dysfunction, poverty, school failure, and early behavior problems—are a promising investment. Finally, there is greater recognition that solutions reside in both the public and private domains—in family relations, popular culture, and public policies.

> "*The ubiquitous media label for teen motherhood, 'children having children'. . . evokes the cultural discomfort the phenomenon stirs, but it's more evocative than accurate.*"

The Media Exaggerate the Problem of Teenage Pregnancy

Janine Jackson

In the following viewpoint, Janine Jackson contends that the media unfairly blame teenage motherhood for causing poverty, which enables policy makers to justify draconian welfare reform. However, according to Jackson, the majority of teen mothers were already poor when they got pregnant. By blaming teenage mothers for economic problems that have complex causes, the mainstream media make it difficult for policy makers to find real solutions to the economic problems that contribute to teenage pregnancy. Janine Jackson is the program director of FAIR (Fairness and Accuracy in Reporting), a national media watch group, and a frequent contributor to its publication *Extra!*

As you read, consider the following questions:
1. As cited by the author, what does Charles Murray consider the "old way, which worked"?
2. What are three disadvantages of teen motherhood, as described by the author?
3. As stated by the author, why do many politicians and members of the media long for "stigma" to be reattached to teenage pregnancy?

From "The 'Crisis' of Teen Pregnancy," by Janine Jackson, *Extra!*, March/April, 1994. Copyright © 1994 by Fairness and Accuracy in Reporting. Reprinted with permission.

A recent round of media attention focused on the "tragedy" of teenage pregnancy, casting the unmarried teenaged mother as the source of virtually all of society's ills. Papers and pundits were moved to florid prose on teen mothers' "world of warped morals and wasted lives that affects the quality of life for all of us." (*Cleveland Plain Dealer*)

Various indicators on birth rates and poverty rates were tossed around to document the "social catastrophe." (*Detroit News*) No serious analysis was needed, since it was obvious to bipartisan politicians and media alike that the "soaring birth rate among welfare mothers" (*Chicago Sun-Times*) is "the smoking gun in a sickening array of pathologies—crime, drug abuse, physical and mental illness, welfare dependency." (*Newsweek*) *USA Today* reported in a near-panic: "Beyond the drugs and the gunfire lies what is perhaps the most shocking of social pathologies: rates of out-of-wedlock births."

The most recent round of finger-pointing was largely touched off by a *Wall Street Journal* op-ed by the American Enterprise Institute's Charles Murray, which contended that "illegitimacy is the single most important social problem of our time—more important than crime, drugs, poverty, illiteracy, welfare or homelessness, because it drives everything else."

Murray's call for denial of all government support to any unmarried woman who has a child (and orphanages for children whose parents can't support them) fits a familiar conservative pattern of blaming poverty on the character faults and bad decisions of the poor themselves. He hearkens back to "the old way, which worked," and calls for making "illegitimate birth the socially horrific act it used to be."

Condemning Unwed Mothers

What was chilling was how easily the mainstream media latched on to Murray's ideology-laden notions, presenting the condemnation of poor unwed mothers as a fresh policy approach—"given the failure of all other remedies." (*Detroit News*)

In fact, the conservative argument's assumptions are demonstrably false, but it successfully plays on cultural (and racial) tensions and fears, along with the need for scapegoats in times of economic strain. Unfortunately, mainstream media have done a poor job of separating moralistic arguments from economic ones.

Journalists speak of "teen pregnancies and the underclass" as "entwined social pathologies." (*Atlanta Journal and Constitution*) But few question *why* this should be.

Substantial evidence shows that while single motherhood is associated with poverty, it does not *cause* poverty. First, most teenagers who give birth were living at or below poverty levels to begin with. Explaining their choice to researchers, these women speak of factors associated with socio-economic status: educational failure, low self-esteem (often connected with sexual abuse) and a lack of job opportunities. These factors, not "the sex-me-up songs on radio and television" (*Plain Dealer*), can make early motherhood appear to be a rational option.

Young Mothers Lack Resources

After becoming mothers, young women are confronted with a lack of affordable childcare and a job market that pays women (especially minority women) inadequate, disproportionately low wages. That many are pushed below the poverty level is not surprising. Nor is it surprising that single fathers are less than half as likely to live in poverty as single mothers.

In an earlier round of the "unwed mothers" discussion, this overlooked economic context was pointed out by family historian Stephanie Coontz in a *Washington Post* op-ed. Most poverty in the U.S., Coontz wrote, is related not to family structure, but to workforce and wage structures, including the "growth of low-wage work that makes one income inadequate to support a family."

"The United States tolerates higher levels of child poverty in *every* family form than any other major industrial democracy," Coontz wrote. "The fastest growing poverty group in America since 1979 has been married-couple families with children."

Nevertheless, the notion that cutting women's welfare benefits will discourage them from having children is finding new receptivity among the press and policymakers, including former president Bill Clinton, who called Murray's idea "essentially right."

"What many experts suspect, and fear," *Newsweek*'s Joe Klein told readers, "is that nothing short of [Murray's] draconian solution . . . will change the culture of chronic dependency." The *Milwaukee Sentinel* called it "the only real way to send the message that illegitimacy doesn't pay."

Real Youth Experiences

Contrary to their negative images, the reality is that most youth do not experience most of the problems reflected in media coverage, such as school failure, drug use, or teen pregnancy. Roughly 20 percent–33 percent of adolescents experience one or more of those problems, for example, and although we would wish for no one to be in that boat, it is hardly sinking; even those levels of malady mean about 66 percent–80 percent of adolescents do not experience those problems. It also should be noted that there is a difference between engaging in *patterns* of high-risk behavior, and one or two instances of experimentation. For example, most young people engage in some form of illegal activity at some time during their adolescent years, but the overwhelming majority does not develop consistent patterns of anti-social behavior, or later turn into career criminals. Indeed, some experimentation with what most adults would call risky behavior seems to be a normal part of adolescent development.

Peter C. Scales, *Society*, May/June 2001.

Murray's basic theory—that women have children because of the "economic incentive" of welfare—has been thoroughly disproven by research, most recently in a study by the Urban Institute (*Urban Institute Policy and Research Report*, Fall/93). The study found that "generosity [of welfare payments] has at best a very modest impact on a woman's initial childbearing decision and virtually no effect on subsequent births."

What did have significant impact, the researchers found, were education, race and income. Fairness and Accuracy in Reporting (FAIR) saw no major media reporting on these findings.

Inaccurate Labels

The ubiquitous media label for teen motherhood, "children having children"—or even "babies having babies," as syndicated columnist Charles Krauthammer put it (*Washington Post*)—evokes the cultural discomfort the phenomenon stirs, but it's more evocative than accurate, since about two-thirds of teenage births are to women 18 and 19, not 13 or 14.

Many welfare rights and women's advocates also believe the "children having children" label infantilizes adolescent mothers, helping to justify policies that treat them as incapable of making decisions. Punitive proposals that compel teenage mothers to live with their families and stay in school in order to receive public assistance (no analogous rules are suggested for fathers) are justified by the press because unwed mothers are, "especially if they're teenagers, plain ignorant." (*New York Times* editorial)

But as Mike Males has pointed out, labeling pregnancies of women under 20 a "teen" problem is itself questionable, since 70 percent of such pregnancies result from sex with a man over 20. Some 50,000 teen pregnancies a year are the result of rape, and two-thirds of teen mothers have a history of rape or sexual molestation, with a perpetrator averaging 27 years of age (*In These Times*). You won't find mention of this in editorials decrying "teenagers shouting about their 'right' to become mothers." (*Plain Dealer*)

Some in the press mourned the loss of the "stigma" of teen pregnancy. *Newsweek* asked, in an interview with President Clinton: "Should we reattach a stigma to those who are having children out of wedlock?" In an *NBC Nightly News* report, Betty Rollin announced, "The stigma of being an unwed mother is history." She then went on to harangue teenage girls about their pregnancies: "Did you feel any shame about this?"

The nostalgia for "stigma" suggests that what many politicians and their supporters in the media find troubling is not so much teen pregnancy as teen sexuality, and that their intention is not so much to offer young women better choices as to socially engineer the "right" kind of families.

Selective Media Exposure

While they hype the urgency of the crisis, mainstream media simultaneously constrict the range of debate, such that simplistic "solutions" crowd out years of relevant research.

Charles Murray was cited in 55 major dailies and newsweeklies in the two months following his *Wall Street Journal* column; his ideas appeared in many more. . . .

On the other hand, social service agencies and research groups that actually work with pregnant teens and young mothers, who might point out the fallacies and omissions in conservative proposals, were largely missing from stories concerned with moralizing and "New Democrat" rhetoric.

Of the many newspaper and magazine articles on the topic of teen pregnancy, only a handful contained comments from actual teen mothers, whose motivations and beliefs are the subject of so much speculation. The object of high-minded harangues and the target of endless programs, their voices are easily drowned out in both the media and the policy debate.

Getting Tough

The talk about Clinton's stand on teenage pregnancy as proof that he [would] "get tough on entitlements" is evidence of another distressing media trend: the tendency to see complex socio-economic issues primarily as political footballs. *Time* magazine confronted President Bill Clinton: "There's a story in the paper saying that the stigma has been removed from teenage pregnancy and that Democrats are responsible."

The *Cleveland Plain Dealer* summed up the significance of welfare "reform" proposals that may disrupt the lives of millions of people: "Riding on the outcome are Clinton's claim to be a 'new Democrat' and the hopes of dozens of moderate and conservative House Democrats hoping to pocket a politically popular vote in time for [the next election]."

By allowing symbolic politics to outweigh reasoned research, and by focusing attention on individual teens and their morals, media accounts of teen pregnancy sidestep just the issues politicians of both parties want to avoid: the role of structural economic forces that condemn single mothers—and many others—to poverty.

> "*Teen moms now go to school, get jobs, get married and, like people of any age, grow into their parenting role.*"

Teenagers Can Make Good Parents

Jasmine Miller

In the following viewpoint, Jasmine Miller describes how teen Shannon Felix proved to the Catholic Children's Aid Society (CCAS) in Canada that her youth and unwed marital status did not preclude her from providing well for her children. Miller argues that unwed teenage pregnancy does not carry the social stigma it used to and that young parents can lead productive, educated lives, even with the burden of an early pregnancy. Jasmine Miller is a contributor to *Chatelaine*, a Canadian-based women's magazine, and was a teenage mother herself.

As you read, consider the following questions:

1. How does Miller describe the stereotype of teenage motherhood?
2. Under what conditions did Shannon Felix get her boys back?
3. According to the author, what high-risk factors do nurses look for in teenage mothers?

Sixteen kids and 20 adults stroll through the kitchen, past huge deep fryers and walk-in freezers and down a flight of narrow stairs to one of a few small party rooms in the basement. Shannon Felix, the mother of the three boys turning three today, freezes. She's forgotten her camera and takes a moment to berate herself. But quickly she's back to orchestrating the event: taking orders from the kids, chatting with guests and moving presents out of the way with one hand while wiping a messy nose or sticky fingers with the other. Her sons, all in matching fleece outfits, sing "Happy birthday to us," take turns on their father's lap and sit wide-eyed and upright when their small cake with thick blue and white icing arrives. It's a '90s Norman Rockwell, the picture of middle-class average. A Sunday afternoon at Playland in a suburban McDonald's.

Hard to believe Shannon's only 19, which makes her the worst kind of stereotype—a teen mom. It's a loaded label that makes no distinction between a married 18-year-old and a 14-year-old dropout. Despite her performance today, Shannon, pregnant at 15 and with three sons at 16, was a conspicuous example of social decay, the demise of the traditional family, one more baby having babies.

Premature Triplets

Before the end of her first trimester, Shannon knew she was having triplets. A Catholic, she'd already made the decision not to abort. "It was my mistake, not theirs," she says. It was a difficult pregnancy. There'd been 10 weeks of bedrest before the C-section seven weeks ahead of her due date. Shannon recovered from the births quickly but the boys stayed in intensive care. Underweight, they were suffering from respiratory and heart problems, consuming all their calories through feeding tubes.

Shannon took public transit for an hour or two to the hospital, depending where she was staying, to be with her sons, sometimes staying overnight, sometimes only for a few hours. At her request, the boys were moved from Women's College Hospital (in downtown Toronto, Canada) to Scarborough Hospital, a 15-minute bus ride from her mother's home. Sheldon, Deon and Keston stayed there for four weeks.

But the temporary nursery Shannon had planned in her mother's apartment would never be set up. The Catholic Children's Aid Society (CCAS) swooped in and put the boys in foster care before they were all discharged. Shannon doesn't have a drug problem. She wasn't a street kid and there was no reason to suspect she'd be abusive or neglectful. She was, however, poor (living off her mother's welfare cheques) and a parent for the first time. There was no chance to prove what kind of mother she would be.

In the end, the organization's swift response to Shannon's situation reflects the pervasive belief about teen mothers. Talk shows are riddled with the stereotype: at its worst, a shiftless irresponsible teen cranking out babies for welfare cheques; at its best, a lonely pathetic girl looking for unconditional love. Good or bad, it's outdated.

Shannon and I have little in common, but I was also a teen mother. And we share the embarrassment and anger this stereotype instills.

Teen Pregnancy Is Increasing

Between 1974 and 1988, the pregnancy rate for Canadians aged 15 to 19 dropped sharply. Although the number has been slowly inching upward since then, teen parenting is not on the rise: more teens are choosing abortion. Only six per cent of live births in 1994 were to teenagers. Still, teen parenting remains high on Canadians' list of social concerns— and for good reason: teen parents are more likely to be poor than their older counterparts, and children who grow up in poverty are at increased risk of just about every negative thing imaginable. Less than ideal circumstances under which to have a baby, for sure, but hardly the automatic ticket to failure it's made out to be.

"Teen parenting is not a permanent state," says Susan Clark, executive director of the Nova Scotia Council on Higher Education, who's been studying parenting since the 1970s. Clark and her team participated in a study initiated by the Department of Community Services in 1978, tracking 700 mothers and their children over the next 20 years.

The second wave of the study, published in 1991, exposed some counterintuitive facts, most notably: the children of younger mothers generally performed within the normal academic range. Teen moms now go to school, get jobs, get married and, like people of any age, grow into their parenting role. More than half of the single teen moms in this study were married by the time their first child was five years old; most continued to be married to the same person while their child was growing up. While most of the single teen moms had less than Grade 12 education at the beginning of the study (76 per cent), by the time their kids were 20 years old, most had finished high school or taken vocational training or other upgrading to help them find jobs.

Researcher Margaret Dechman is heading up the third wave of the study "Even by the time of the 10-year data collection," she says from her Halifax office, "some of the notions of teen mothers simply weren't [accurate]." Far from creating a generational cycle of dependence, the average single teenage mother spent only three years on welfare before her child was 10 years old. The point of all this research? Life doesn't stop at adolescence, even for people who start families before we think they should.

CCAS Steps In

On Nov. 21, 1996, Shannon arrived at the maternity ward of Scarborough Hospital with her mother and the boys' father, Rodney Mayers, to see her sons. A hospital social worker told her they would be going to foster care instead. The CCAS was worried about Shannon's housing arrangements: the one-bedroom apartment she shared with her mother was too small. When Shannon, in her own words, "lost it," she was told she also had an anger-management problem. At the first custody hearing, the CCAS changed its stance: Shannon's truancy record proved she wasn't responsible enough for parenthood.

"The woman they gave my kids to," Shannon says, referring to the foster parent chosen by the CCAS, "was, like, 60 years old. No one ever mentioned it, but I know that was the biggest reason. It was because of my age."

Shannon is close to 10 years younger than I am, grew up in public housing and dropped out of school at an age when I was looking forward to French immersion and class trips to

Montreal. But I was 17 and one credit shy of a high school diploma when I got pregnant. I'd been dating my boyfriend for about two years and had stopped taking the pill because of some random symptoms my doctor said could be attributed to the pastel discs I'd popped diligently for months. With a confidence unique to teenagers, I took my chances, believing that if I didn't want to get pregnant, I wouldn't. I wasn't using any birth control when I conceived.

I'm not religious; I can't say why I never considered abortion. Like most pregnant teens, I immediately dismissed adoption as a possibility. I had a plan: a day-care subsidy and a student loan, a university degree and then a job. My counsellor at the health clinic wasn't impressed or optimistic. The last time I saw her, she pressed into my sweaty hand a doctor's card and an information package on dilation and curettage [scraping the walls of the uterus].

Teenage Sexuality

By getting pregnant, teenagers accost us with their sexuality. While we talk open-mindedly about the need for teens to be educated about sex and its repercussions, our stomachs turn when we're presented with proof of their maturity. I knew I had let my family down, that family friends would whisper about what a shame it was and blame my absent father and liberal mother for my downfall. At 18, I became the first person in my family ever to collect welfare. I don't think much was expected of me after that—I'd already messed up as much as a young girl could.

"We have rigid notions of what we think teens should be doing," says Margaret McKinnon, dean of the faculty of education at the University of Regina, who is part of a research team that develops programs to get teen moms back into the classroom. "We think they should be in school getting a good education to get a good job. What I ask is, 'Are we ensuring that that is in fact what all teens can expect?'" McKinnon thinks we're falling short on that front, and if we don't give teens alternatives, then "Having a baby can make a lot of good sense." She's not advocating teen parenting, though, and she's not looking for an answer when she asks, "Without choices, why not have a baby now?"

McKinnon's explanation, though charitable, makes me uneasy. Accepting it means believing the decision to have a baby is usually deliberate; that only girls from poor families or those who have little ambition find themselves pregnant as teenagers. But that wasn't the case with Shannon—motherhood was not on her agenda back then. At 15, she was hanging out at the mall, thinking about the next party and skipping classes. "I could kick myself in the butt," she says. "I would have been in college by now, but everyone's got to make their mistakes and learn from them."

Shannon invited me to her place, a tidy three-bedroom bungalow on a treelined street. She's no stranger to journalists: in the middle of her fight to get her kids back, her brother blitzed the local media with phone calls. The nose ring she wore when her picture was all over the papers is gone, but standing in her doorway in baggy khakis and a sweater, Shannon looks younger than she is. She also looks tired but smiles at her sons, who are jumping around, performing for this surprise visitor.

Fighting Back

I'm trying to find out what happened next, what she felt that morning when the nurse told her the boys were with a foster family but refused to tell her where that family lived. Shannon's answer is to show me all the papers. There's the certificate she earned for completing the Nobody's Perfect Parenting Program—a condition of getting the kids back and, according to Shannon, a waste of time. "We ate pizza and made playdough. You can't teach parenting." There are also three copies of each affidavit, notice of hearing, protection application and court transcript in a three-ring binder. "I kept them to show the boys that I wouldn't leave them," she says, dropping the stack with a thud beside me.

Since Shannon was a minor when she gave birth, the CCAS had to pay a lawyer to represent her in her custody battle. That lawyer can't talk about the case. The lawyer for the CCAS can't talk about it either (in accordance with the Child and Family Services Act) and won't return calls, but a message on his voice mail earned me a call from the agency's public relations department and the promise of a followup call. It's been a year. In the end, there's just Shannon's side of the story and a paper trail.

In the court documents, the official explanation is this: "The apprehension of the children was based on the society's need to further assess the mother's plan for the children, her parenting capacity, her willingness to co-operate with services . . . and her ability to meet the demands of three premature infants." A month after the boys left the hospital, a family court judge decided Shannon could take them home— but under CCAS supervision.

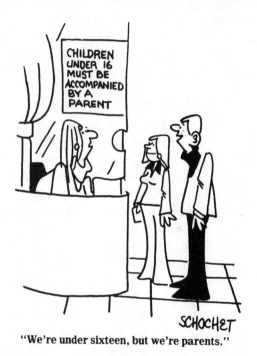

"We're under sixteen, but we're parents."

Schochet. © 1987 by the *Wall Street Journal*. Reprinted with permission.

There were conditions: Shannon would have to move in with her aunt, uncle and cousins in their four-bedroom house. She would agree to unannounced visits by social workers. At the second home visit the social worker wrote that "The mother has embraced motherhood with commitment and devotion." On Dec. 20, 1996, Shannon was awarded full custody of her sons. "I hate what they did to us," she says of the CCAS.

Shannon recalls it was Sheila Neubeurger, a patient care worker at the Scarborough Hospital, who made that first phone call to the Children's Aid Society. Although Neubeurger can't talk specifically about the case, she discussed the "social high-risk factors" nurses look for: "No prenatal care or inconsistent prenatal care, a history of drug or alcohol use, a history of sexual or physical abuse. If there's nobody around, if the only other person you see is another 15-year-old. . . ." Pretty quickly, I'm reminded of Shannon's life, even though Neubeurger could just as easily be talking about a 35-year-old as a 16-year-old mother. "Teens who dropped out when they were 12 and when you ask, they haven't been doing much. Lack of housing, lack of finances." The worker sums up pregnancy in adolescence this way: "It doesn't go with that stage of life."

Creating Their Family

Shannon and Rodney, five years her senior, don't live together and they have no plans to marry ("I'm too young for that," Shannon tells me, oblivious to any irony). But they are a couple and a family—Rodney has always been a disciplinarian and playmate to his sons.

"Who flies the planes?" Shannon asks the two boys who are belted into the back seat. "The pilot!" the toddlers scream in unison, squirming with laughter. Deon is strapped into the front seat, beside his father. "Deon, I told you not to touch the wheel," Rodney tells him for the third time.

Back home, all three of the boys are at the kitchen table eating fistfuls of Cheerios while Shannon gets dinner ready. It's organized chaos. Sheldon has stripped down to his underwear and Deon is standing on his chair, something he knows is not allowed. Bedtime is 8 P.M. Two hours later, the giggling requests for juice and kisses have finally stopped; there's a late movie on TV and Shannon's folding another load of laundry.

There's no way of knowing if Shannon's kids would have been better off with a 40-year-old parent or if Shannon would have been better off waiting till 40 to become one. We make a lot of assumptions about teen mothers. We figure 30-

year-olds can cope with parenthood and that 16-year-olds can't. We think teen parents will be on welfare forever and their kids won't have much hope of a better life—and the whole thing will repeat itself.

At 28, I still haven't been able to shake the "teen mom" label. If I hadn't succumbed to the stereotype, would I have a master's degree and not just a BA? Would I have a better job than the one that covers my mortgage now? When the school calls to tell me that my son got into a fight or bombed a math test, I can't help but wonder if that's at least part of the reason. Would Calvin be better off if I'd had him at 35? Or even 21?

Shannon is now working toward finishing her high school diploma with plans to study computers or engineering in college. "I have to make enough to get off the system," she says. Maybe she's dreaming; maybe she'll change her mind or just not make it. Whatever the case, for Shannon and for me, motherhood was an inspiration. It's hard to predict a right or wrong time for that.

"I can't picture my life without them," Shannon tells me. "I can't say I wish I'd waited till I finished high school and got married because I probably wouldn't have gotten this far if I didn't have them."

> *"If a teen [decides] to have a baby he or she has the [responsibility] to look after it, take care of it, love it, and give it shelter."*

Teenage Parents Face Daunting Challenges

Lisa W.

In the following viewpoint, high school student Lisa W. argues that teen pregnancy and childbearing present difficult challenges. She maintains that many teenage mothers fail to complete their education and end up on welfare. Moreover, the children of teenage parents are often born with birth defects and later suffer behavioral problems.

As you read, consider the following questions:
1. According to the author, how are boys commonly affected by their mother's teenage pregnancy?
2. What should teenage parents teach their own children about adolescent sex and pregnancy, as stated by the author?
3. According to the author, why are many teenagers' babies born premature?

T een pregnancy is very common all over the world.
Teens from the ages of ten to nineteen years old are having babies. In a sense, babies are having babies. Pregnancy and giving birth to a child is a very big responsibility. Many teens that become pregnant have abortions, put their babies up for adoption, or just do not take care of them at all. Is it right for teens to be getting pregnant at such a young age? Why is this happening in our society where there is so much education available? These are questions that are asked throughout the world.

How Bad Is the Problem?

The United States has the highest rates of teen pregnancy and births in the world. Four out of ten young women become pregnant at least once before they reach the age of twenty. Eight out of ten of these pregnancies are unintended.

The teen birth rate declined 18 percent from 1991 to 1998 for teens aged fifteen to nineteen. It is said that the younger a teenage girl is when she has sexual intercourse for the first time, the more likely she is to have had unwanted or non-voluntary sexual intercourse. Close to four out of ten girls who had intercourse at thirteen or fourteen years of age [claim that the sex] was either non-voluntary or unwanted.

The person who suffers the consequences the most are the teen mothers themselves. Teen mothers are less likely to complete and graduate high school and more likely to end up on welfare [than teen girls who wait to have babies]. If they give the baby up, when they grow older they are more likely to be sorry for giving their babies up and want them back.

Studies have shown that sons of teen mothers are thirteen percent more likely to end up in prison, while teen daughters are twenty-two percent more likely to become teen mothers themselves.

Young teens who have babies should ensure that, when their baby grows up, they teach him/her not to make the same mistake that they did. They should tell them to wait until they are ready to have sex, and have a partner that they know they will be with for a very long time. It is definitely not necessary for teens to become pregnant at such a young age.

How Can Teen Pregnancy Be Prevented?

Teen pregnancy can be prevented in many ways. Some of the reasons given as to why some teen girls do not get pregnant or have sex at an early age are: its against their religious or moral values; they don't want to get sexually transmitted diseases or haven't met an appropriate partner. Three out of four girls say that they only have sexual intercourse because their boyfriends want them to.

The Costs of Teenage Pregnancy

Despite the decline in birth rates for teens, the problem of teenage pregnancy remains serious in the United States. The number of sexually active teens has increased, causing the overall pregnancy rates to increase. Every 26 seconds another adolescent becomes pregnant, and every 56 seconds another adolescent gives birth. Today, adolescent pregnancy continues to be a multidimensional problem that has staggering social and economic tolls on individuals, families, and communities within the American society. The profound impact is evident in the physical, psychosocial, and cognitive development of the mother and infant and reaches beyond the price of diapers and formula to the price of shattered families and unrealized dreams. Usually, pregnancies of young, unmarried women have the following outcomes:

- 50% of these pregnancies will end in abortion.
- 43% will end in an unintentional birth.
- 7% will end as an intended birth.

Donna Wong, *Wong on Web*, 1999.

Many teens who have already had sexual intercourse, including boys and girls, say they wish they could have waited. This is because doing such activity at a young age could more than likely ruin your life. Many babies that are being born today grow up not having a father. One reason for this is because the mothers are promiscuous, and have no idea who the father could be. Another reason is that the fathers don't want the responsibility of taking care of their babies so they run away from their responsibilities and most times never come back.

Many babies are being born premature. "Why?" is a question that some people ask. This is because the mothers do not take care of their own bodies. Some of this leads to babies dying. Babies die because of a lot of reasons. Some of these reasons may include having diseases such as H.I.V. Babies also die of a disease called Fetal Alcohol Syndrome. Fetal Alcohol Syndrome is a disease that infants can get if their mothers drink heavily during the pregnancy.

This disease can lead to death or serious health problems. Sometimes, when babies are born with this disease they get a hole in their heart and surgery has to be performed on them immediately. Babies may also get diseases from drugs that their parents used during pregnancy or intercourse. Low birth weight of a baby doubles the chances that a child will have some kind of disability. Although these are the most common reasons for children being born premature, there are many, many more.

An Enormous Responsibility

In my opinion, teen pregnancy is not right and can be prevented. A teen should know the responsibilities of having a child and how [teenage childbearing] affects the life of the baby and themselves. If a teen [decides] to have a baby he or she has the [responsibility] to look after it, take care of it, love it, and give it shelter. They created the baby so they should live with the consequences and difficulties of taking care of it and being a parent.

Periodical Bibliography

The following articles have been selected to supplement the diverse views presented in this chapter.

Alan Guttmacher Institute	"Why Is Teenage Pregnancy Declining? The Roles of Abstinence, Sexual Activity, and Contraceptive Use," 1999.
Jimmie Briggs	"Where Have All the Babies Gone?" *Family Planning Life*, January 1998.
Maggie Gallagher	"Hollow Victory on Teen Pregnancy," *Conservative Chronicle*, November 10, 1999.
Farrah M. McDaid	"Tribal Teen Pregnancies Raise Red Flags," *California Journal*, May 1, 2000.
Randall K. O'Bannon	"Latest CDC Data Show U.S. Abortion Rate Holding Steady," *National Right to Life News*, December 10, 1998.
William Petersen	"Age and Sex," *Society*, May/June 2001.
Isabel V. Sawhill	"Teen Pregnancy Prevention: Welfare Reform's Missing Component," *Brookings Policy Brief*, November 1998.
Peter C. Scales	"The Public Image of Adolescents," *Society*, May/June 2001.
Oliver Starr Jr.	"Teen Girls Are Easy Prey for Over-20 Predators," *Insight on the News*, May 3, 1999.
Emory Thomas Jr.	"Is Pregnancy a Rational Choice for Poor Teenagers?" *Wall Street Journal*, January 18, 1996.
Stephanie J. Ventura and Sally C. Curtin	"Recent Trends in Teen Births in the United States," *Statistical Bulletin*, January–March 1999.
Cheryl Wetzstein and Matthew Katz	"Further Erosion of Marriage Is Expected After Millennium," *Insight on the News*, February 1, 1999.

CHAPTER 2

What Factors Contribute to Teenage Pregnancy?

Chapter Preface

Many cultures consider large age differences between men and women in romantic relationships acceptable. Western culture has traditionally encouraged relationships between young women and older men for two reasons. First, older men often have more financial resources and are better providers than younger men. Second, young women are more likely to produce healthy children than older women.

Many social commentators have argued that this trend encourages adult men to form sexual relationships with underage girls and increase their risk of pregnancy. According to author Linda Villarosa, "67 percent of teenage mothers are impregnated by men who are over twenty years old. . . . Whether coerced or voluntary, couplings between teenage girls and adult males are many times more likely to result in pregnancy than teen-teen sex." Villarosa and others maintain that "predatory" adult males pursue young girls and contribute to the problem of teenage pregnancy.

Others argue that research data that blame significantly older men for the majority of teenage pregnancies has been misinterpreted. According to the Urban Institute, 62 percent of teen pregnancies (births to fifteen- to nineteen-year-olds) involve eighteen- or nineteen-year-old mothers. Moreover, only 27 percent of children born to girls who are fifteen, sixteen, or seventeen are fathered by men at least five years older. The institute found that of teenage pregnancies involving unmarried women aged fifteen to seventeen, only 8 percent were fathered by men who were at least five years older and only 13 percent were fathered by men at least four years older. Some people argue that these data reflect the fact that most teenage mothers are not the youthful victims of older male predators. Instead, most are over the age of 18 and in relationships with men who are less than five years older than they are. As stated by journalist Catherine Elton, "There are clearly cases in which relationships between older men and younger women are inappropriate, but determining which relationships fall into that category requires moral judgments about which Americans are sincerely, and deeply, divided."

> *"Teenage mothers with much-older partners are disproportionately the childhood victims of sexual assault by adult men."*

Older Men Contribute to Teenage Pregnancy

Part I: Linda Valdez; Part II: Ellen Goodman

In the following two-part viewpoint, Linda Valdez and Ellen Goodman argue that adult men take advantage of teenage girls and contribute to the problem of teenage pregnancy. In Part I, Linda Valdez, an editorial columnist, contends that some older men prey on vulnerable young girls who are looking for a male role model. In Part II, Ellen Goodman claims that recent legislative action revived statutory rape laws, which were largely ignored during the sexual revolution and women's movement. Valdez and Goodman agree that enforcing statutory rape laws can protect young girls from exploitation by older men and reduce the incidence of teenage pregnancy. Goodman is a columnist for the *Boston Globe*.

As you read, consider the following questions:
1. According to Valdez, why do many young girls seek a male role model?
2. What precipitated renewed interest in statutory rape laws, according to Goodman?
3. According to Goodman, why were statutory rape laws abandoned during the sexual revolution and the women's movement?

Part I: From "Men and Girls: A Time for Anger," by Linda Valdez, *Masthead*, Fall 1997. Copyright © 1997 by National Conference of Editorial Writers. Reprinted with permission. Part II: From "Teenage Girls Shouldn't Be 'Fair Game,'" by Ellen Goodman, *San Francisco Chronicle*, 1996. Copyright © 1996 by *San Francisco Chronicle*. Reprinted with permission.

I

Grown men who molest very little girls are universally despised. So why doesn't society cast its collective condemnation at grown men who seduce little teenage girls?

Why do we continue to blame a lack of teenage morals for rising rates of teen pregnancy, even though most of the teens who get pregnant are the victims of something we used to call statutory rape?

According to the Arizona Department of Health Services, 66.3% of babies born to teenage girls in 1994 were fathered by men age 20 or older.

The Washington Alliance Concerned With School Age Parents conducted a survey in Seattle of mothers ages 12 to 17 in 1995 and found the average age of the fathers was 24.

An article in the *American Journal of Public Health* in the spring of 1997 cited statistics for California's teen mothers. In 1993, wrote authors Mike Males and Kenneth S.Y. Chew, two-thirds of school-age teen mothers had a post-school-age partner.

A 15-year-old girl does not have the experience or emotional sophistication to match wits with a 20-year-old man. She might be conned into having sex, but she is incapable of giving consent.

Legal Protection

Society used to understand that. Laws against having sex with underage girls were enforced. Men understood that these children were off limits. Communities did not wink as 25-year-old men escorted 17-year-old girls to the prom.

These days laws against statutory rape—now known by the euphemism "sexual conduct with a minor"—are not enforced.

Prosecution is difficult and the girls are reluctant to testify. These days men are not afraid of the consequences of going after young girls. These days communities do wink when girls show up with men at the prom.

The reasons girls go with older men are complex and relatively unexplored.

According to Males and Chew: "The [age] gap is especially significant because teenage mothers with much-older partners are disproportionately the childhood victims of sexual assault by adult men. The possibility that much early childbearing represents an extension of rape or sexual abuse by male perpetrators averaging one to two decades older remains a serious question."

According to the U.S. Justice Department, females under 18 are the victims of half the rapes committed in this country each year.

Even if they are not being physically intimidated, young girls are easy prey to emotional appeals from older men. Divorce and single parenthood has left many girls hungry for a strong male model.

"You can only speculate what this is replacing," says Billie Enz, Arizona State professor and expert on teen pregnancy. "They're looking for a father image that they can fall in love with. You have to wonder about the man that would take advantage of that situation."

And you have to wonder about people—from parents to legislators to teachers—who would look the other way while those men hunt their prey unencumbered by social condemnation and the serious threat of jail time.

II

You could say that politics makes strange bedfellows, but bedfellows is probably not the best word to use considering the subject. The subject is sex, teenage pregnancy, welfare—a trio of issues that have morphed into public enemy number one. An enemy with a face that is young and female.

In the past, politicians outdid each other in their praise of motherhood. Today they outdo each other in laments about teenage motherhood. From the feminist left to the religious right, they have found common ground worrying and sermonizing over girls who become mothers before they become women.

Now at last, the same disparate collection of policy-makers are turning their attention to the partners in this terrible tango: adult men.

Bringing Back Statutory Rape

In California, which has the highest rate of teenage pregnancy in the country, former governor Pete Wilson, who tacked from right to center with impressive sailing skills, issued a warning to adult men who impregnate underage girls. In his state of the state address in January 1996, he told these men, "I have this message: That's not just wrong, not just a shame. It's a crime, a crime called statutory rape."

Predatory Older Men

The exploitation of teenage girls by older men may be one of the nation's most serious social problems, but it seldom is written or talked about. Approximately 900,000 teenage girls become pregnant each year; a little more than half of them give birth. The conventional wisdom is that their classmates father nearly all of these children. But a 1992 California Department of Health Services study showed that more than three-quarters of these children were fathered by men older than 20 and more than 70 percent of the births were out of wedlock. The study further found that men older than 20 also father five times more births among junior-high-school girls than do junior-high-school boys.

Oliver Starr Jr., *Insight on the News*, May 3, 1999.

Wilson allotted $150,000 to each of 16 counties to go after men who go after girls. It's an idea whose time has come back. And not just in California.

The renewed interest in statutory rape laws comes out of startling research showing that the babies of teenage moms don't necessarily have teenage dads. Half the babies born to mothers between 15 and 17 had fathers who were over 20.

Across the country, 20 percent of the fathers are six or more years older than the mothers. The younger the girl, the greater the age difference.

You do the math. Former president Bill Clinton's National Campaign to Reduce Teen Pregnancy wants to cut teen pregnancy by a third by 2005. Half the impregnators are adult men. Any rational discussion of this issue has to include these men.

Young Girls Should Be Off Limits

In California, one of Wilson's goals was, surely, to collect child support money by threatening imprisonment. But the other goal is to post a protective sign—"Off Limits"—

around young and vulnerable girls. This is where the support for dusting off these laws is growing—out of a concern about exploitation and abuse, sexual pressure and predators.

In early America, the age of consent for a girl was 10. Then in the 19th century, a movement made up of feminists and moralists and reformers of many stripes raised the age as high as 18 or 20 for the explicit purpose of protecting young females and their "virtues" from men and their "vices."

But a generation ago, in the wake of the sexual revolution and the women's movement, the social pendulum swung from protecting females to liberating them. Statutory rape laws seemed to stereotype both sexes while giving the state the right to decide who could and couldn't consent to sex.

Most of the laws were put into mothballs. As a result, Michelle Oberman of DePaul University says, "Modern criminal law has turned girls from 'jail bait' to 'fair game'."

Now, in many ways, we are concerned again that we have abandoned the responsibility to children. In the real world, "liberation" left girls more vulnerable, and the reform did little to right the power imbalance of age and gender.

I'm not in favor of these laws if they are used to prosecute the 18-year-old boyfriends of 17-year-old girls. Every 17-year-old girl is not a victim. Nor is every 18-year-old boy a predator. But this is one way for society to draw a line. This is one way for society to right the power imbalance. It's time to say again that adolescent girls are not "fair game."

"Births to minors and older men constitute a relatively small proportion of all teenage childbearing."

Older Men May Not Contribute to Teenage Pregnancy

Laura Duberstein Lindberg, Freya L. Sonenstein, Leighton Ku, and Gladys Martinez

Recent studies have suggested that relationships between adult males and teenage girls account for about two-thirds of adolescent pregnancies. However, these men are usually less than five years older than the mother, which may show that the relationships are consensual. In the following viewpoint, Laura Duberstein Lindberg, Freya L. Sonenstein, Leighton Ku, and Gladys Martinez contend that while adult men father some adolescent pregnancies, most teenage parents are closer in age than previously thought. Lindberg and Martinez are research associates, Ku is a senior research associate, and Sonenstein is the director, all at the Urban Institute, a nonpartisan economic and social policy research organization.

As you read, consider the following questions:
1. According to the authors, which group of girls was most likely to have a partner five or more years older?
2. What kind of relationships did the authors find existed between teenage girls and their older partners?
3. What policies do the authors suggest to reduce the number of teenage pregnancies?

During the last decade, researchers began questioning the assumption that the sexual partners of teenage mothers were necessarily teenagers themselves. Recently, studies have indicated that a majority of babies born to teenage girls were fathered by adult men. Public attention has become focused on the role of "predatory" adult men in teenage childbearing. This view has led some states, such as California and Florida, to toughen and expand their statutory rape laws. In addition, the 1996 federal welfare reform laws specified, as a strategy to reduce teenage pregnancy, "that States and local jurisdictions should aggressively enforce statutory rape laws."

While prior research made important contributions showing that adult males father many of the children of adolescent mothers, such studies have tended to treat teenage mothers and their adult partners as a homogenous group. Although D.J. Landry and J.D. Forrest provided a number of measures of age-gaps between fathers and mothers, often just one combination is cited—that of mothers aged 15–19 with partners aged 20 or older; in their study, 65% of 15–19-year-old mothers had a partner aged 20 or older. M. Males and K.S.Y. Chew took a similar conceptual approach, identifying "school-aged" mothers (ages 10–18) and their non-school-aged partners (19 or older).

Grouping together 15–19-year-olds and their partners ages 20 and older may misrepresent the issue of adolescents bearing children with older men. First, regardless of the mother's age, the pattern of fathers being slightly older than mothers fits squarely within societal norms. For example, in 1988, babies born to women aged 21–30 were fathered by men who were, on average, three years older than their partner. While a 25-year-old man fathering a child with a 15-year-old would probably meet with social disapproval, the same might not be true for a couple consisting of a 21-year-old and an 18-year-old, particularly if they were married.

Second, many relationships between men 20 or older and women 19 or younger do not violate any state's law, provided there is no forcible rape or incest. Although statutory rape laws vary from state to state, they always pertain only to minors—individuals younger than age 18, but the age threshold is lower in many states. Further, most states specify a minimum age that the "perpetrator" must be to be charged or specify a minimum age difference between the partners. . . .

Statutory Rape Laws

Statutory rape laws are not uniformly enforced, however. Although such laws have had a long history in the United States, they had fallen into disuse in the last few decades, and only recently have some states revived and expanded these laws as part of efforts to reduce teenage pregnancy and related public welfare costs. For example, California's Teenage Pregnancy Prevention Act of 1995 created harsh penalties for statutory rape that results in pregnancy. Furthermore, the act earmarks special state funds to expand the prosecution of adult men who father children with minors.

In this article, we present data that examine closely the role of older men in teenage childbearing. To more accurately reflect the policy issues, we limit our analysis to mothers aged 15–17. (Comparable data for mothers aged 14 and younger were unavailable.) In addition, we focus on young women whose partner was at least five years older; such men are referred to as "older" partners throughout. This five-year age difference approximates the typical legal criterion for statutory rape in the five largest states, although other states may use stricter or looser criteria.

Using this five-year definition of age differences between 15–17-year-olds and their partners, we examine three related questions: What is the frequency with which children of 15–17-year-olds are fathered by older men? Second, what are the characteristics of these minors and of their relationships? Finally, how do the socio-economic characteristics of the older men who father children with minors differ from those of other adult fathers, and from those of younger fathers? . . .

How Many Minors?

As expected, conclusions about the role of adult men in adolescent childbearing are sensitive to how the behavior is defined; much of the discussion on the issue has been framed in terms of partners who are at least 20 years old. However, the proportion of 15–17-year-old mothers in 1988 whose partner was at least five years older was substantially lower than the proportion whose partner was at least age 20 (27% vs. 50%). The proportion with at least a five-year age difference among these younger women is not significantly different from that among women aged 18–30.

The youngest mothers in the sample were the most likely to have a partner five or more years older (40%). (By definition, the same proportion had a partner at least 20 years of age.) This proportion dropped to 27% and 24% among 16- and 17-year-olds, respectively. Thus, births to the youngest mothers were disproportionately fathered by much older men who had engaged in sex nine months earlier with 14- and 15-year-olds. On the other hand, births to 15-year-olds made up only 13% of all births to 15–17-year-old women. They thus contribute relatively little to the overall incidence of minors having children fathered by older men.

Births to minors and older men constitute a relatively small proportion of all teenage childbearing. Births to women aged 15–19 can be categorized by the mother's age, the relative age of her partner, and her marital status at the child's birth. The majority of births to women aged 15–19 were to mothers aged 18 or 19 (62%). Births to 15–17-year-olds thus made up only about one-third of all teenage childbearing. Relatively few of these minors were unmarried and had a substantially older male partner: Overall, among all births to 15–19-year-olds in 1988, only 8% involved unmarried women aged 15–17 and men who were at least five years older.

Which Minors?

If births to teenagers result from older men "preying" on young women, then we would expect the most vulnerable among them to be more likely to bear a child with an older man. For example, poverty or other negative home situations may lead young women to look to an adult man for rescue or escape. An alternative explanation, based on problem behavior theory, suggests that minors who engage in risky behavior are more likely to have an older partner, since problem behavior can indicate underlying psychosocial problems and, thus, increased vulnerability. In addition, having sexual relations and a child with an older partner can itself be defined as problem behavior, and problem behaviors often occur together or are correlated with one another.

Two small, nonrepresentative studies found some evidence of a correlation between economic vulnerability and older partners, and between problem behavior and older partners. A study of 300 couples found that teenage mothers who were involved with older men (at least three and one-half years older) were more likely than their peers with similar-age partners to come from poor households, and were more likely to engage in problem behavior. D. Boyer and D. Fine found that teenage mothers who reported having been sexually abused—and who, on average, had older partners—were more likely than nonabused teenage mothers to report a problem behavior, including alcohol and drug use and dropping out of school.

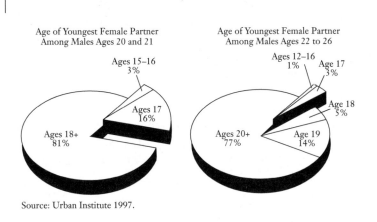

Source: Urban Institute 1997.

Freya L. Sonenstein et al., "Involving Males in Preventing Teen Pregnancy: A Guide for Program Planners," Urban Institute, January 1998.

Contrary to our expectations, the National Maternal and Infant Health Survey (NMIHS) data (1988–1991) show that having an older partner was not strongly associated with the minor's race or household income. Mothers aged 15–17 who lived in the poorest households during their pregnancy (those with a yearly household income of less than $10,000) were marginally less likely than teenage mothers living in higher income households to have had an older partner. One possible confounding factor is that older partners were more likely than similar-age partners to be cohabiting with the mother during the pregnancy, which could raise her household income.

Involvement in problem behavior, however, strongly differentiated minors with older partners from those with similar-age partners. For example, teenage mothers who had already had a child were more likely than those with a first birth to have had an older partner (42% vs. 25%). Furthermore, mothers aged 15–17 who had used alcohol in the three months before the pregnancy were nearly twice as likely to have had an older partner as were those who did not use alcohol (43% vs. 22%).

What Kind of Relationships?

If the relationships between older men and minors are predatory, they might be more casual or transient than those between similar-age partners. In the most extreme cases, babies fathered by older men may be the result of involuntary sexual activity. Alternatively, if older men are viewed as providing a way out of poverty or other undesirable home situations, adolescents may be more likely to establish close relationships with these older men, who potentially have more economic resources available to them than younger men.

Our data indicate that childbearing occurs within the context of ongoing close relationships for an important proportion of 15–17-year-old mothers who have older partners. First, 23% of these young mothers were married at the time they delivered their baby. Thus, overall, 21% of births to unmarried minors were fathered by a much older man. Moreover, 35% of minors with an older partner had been cohabiting during the pregnancy, and 49% were living with their partner at the time of the interview (held up to 30 months after the birth).

The relationships between 15–17-year-old mothers and their older partners appear to be closer than those their peers have with similar-age partners. Although the likelihood of being married at delivery was not significantly different between young mothers with older and similar-age partners, the living arrangements of these young women differed significantly by the age of their partner. Mothers with an older partner were significantly more likely than those with a similar-age partner to have cohabitated during the pregnancy and to be doing so at the time of the interview.

Consequently, adolescent mothers with an older partner were significantly less likely than those with a similar-age partner to have lived with their parents during the pregnancy. Teenage mothers with an older partner were also marginally more likely than those with a similar-age partner to report their pregnancy as wanted, although clearly the majority of births to minors, regardless of their partners' age, were unwanted.

Are Older Men Better Partners?

Young women's economic vulnerability suggests that for some, older men may be more desirable partners than teenage men. On the one hand, older men's age and experience suggest that their immediate earning potential may be greater than that of younger men. On the other hand, an older man involved in a sexual and childbearing relationship with a minor may possess developmental or psychosocial deficits that directly reduce his earning potential and other aspects of his attractiveness as a partner.

Research based on nonrepresentative samples supports both of these hypotheses. In one study, for example, older fathers reported more problem behavior than similar-age fathers, including more arrests and poorer academic performance; however, older fathers also reported higher incomes and employment rates than similar-age fathers. Overall, from the perspective of a teenage woman who is looking for a partner, men in their 20s may appear more "economically desirable"—or, according to [scholar] William Julius Wilson's theories, more "marriageable"—than males who are still teenagers. . . .

Although racial background may be related to lower wage-earning potential, older partners did not differ significantly from similar-age partners by race. However, older fathers were marginally more likely not to have finished high school than similar-age fathers were to be at least two years behind in school (33% vs. 25%). This finding supports the finding of other studies that older partners are more likely than similar-age partners to have engaged in problem behavior. . . .

A Small Percentage

While much recent public attention has focused on the role of adult men in adolescent childbearing, our analyses suggest that this attention has overestimated the extent of the problem for a number of reasons. First, the problem is usually framed in terms of the two-thirds of 15–19-year-olds who have had a child with a man aged 20 and older; the problem is considerably smaller when only mothers who have not reached the age of majority are considered. Second, focusing on fathers who are substantially older than the 15–17-year-old mother—at least five years—also reduces the numbers involved. Third, nearly one-quarter (23%) of minors who have a child with a much older partner are married at the time of the infant's birth. Thus, 21% of births to unmarried minors are fathered by substantially older men. . . .

That births to unmarried minors who have substantially older partners represent a relatively small portion of all U.S. adolescent births belies the popular perception that preventing sexual involvement between older men and young adolescents will substantially reduce rates of teenage pregnancy. New state and federal initiatives that emphasize the vigorous enforcement of statutory rape laws are unlikely to be the magic bullet to reduce rates of adolescent childbearing, since the number of births that result from acts covered by such laws is small. Policymakers need to pay attention to broader means of reducing teenage childbearing, such as sexuality education, youth development and contraceptive services. Policies that improve young women's current lives and expand their future options might better address the issues that lead some to prematurely engage in childbearing and other adult behaviors.

Finally, those few adult men who become involved with considerably younger women may respond to incentives and disincentives to fathering a child with a minor. The disincentives, such as expanding the reach and increasing the penalties of statutory rape laws, have already been advanced; improving access to economic opportunities and achievement for disadvantaged men may be an equally important avenue to try to discourage adult sexual involvement and childbearing with minors.

| *"Sexual abuse [is] strongly associated with adolescent pregnancy."*

Sexual Abuse Contributes to Teenage Pregnancy

Jacqueline L. Stock, Michelle A. Bell, Debra K. Boyer, and Frederick A. Connell

In the following viewpoint, Jacqueline L. Stock, Michelle A. Bell, Debra K. Boyer, and Frederick A. Connell argue that young girls who have been sexually abused are at higher risk for adolescent pregnancy than girls who have not been abused. They maintain that girls who were sexually abused as children manifest high-risk sexual behaviors, such as promiscuity and unprotected sex, which put them at risk for unplanned adolescent pregnancy. Stock is a research study manager at Battelle Centers for Public Health Research. Bell is an associate professor at the University of Washington, Seattle. Boyer is an affiliate associate professor at University of Washington, Seattle. Connell is a professor of maternal and child health services at the University of Washington, Seattle.

As you read, consider the following questions:
1. What are three consequences of sexual abuse, as described by the authors?
2. According to the authors, why do "premature and coercive sexual experiences" put teens at risk for an adolescent pregnancy?
3. How does participation in extracurricular activities factor into teenage pregnancy, according to the authors?

Excerpted from "Adolescent Pregnancy and Sexual Risk-Taking Among Sexually Abused Girls," by Jacqueline L. Stock, Michelle A. Bell, Debra K. Boyer, and Frederick A. Connell, *Family Planning Perspectives*, August/September 1997. Copyright © 1997 by Alan Guttmacher Institute. Reprinted with permission.

As sexual abuse of female children and adolescent pregnancy have gained increasingly widespread public recognition as problems in our society, the relationship between early abuse and teenage pregnancy also has become a focus of attention. However, differences in definitions of abuse, methods of inquiry and study populations have led to discrepant conclusions.

Some studies of adolescent mothers and pregnant adolescents have documented a high prevalence of sexual abuse, ranging from 43% to 62%. However, other studies of pregnant teenagers have reported a sexual abuse prevalence of 15–26%, rates no higher than those most commonly reported for the general population of women.

Whereas data on a small group of college women suggested that those who had been sexually abused were at no higher risk for early pregnancy than their peers who had not been abused, findings from a population-based sample indicated that women who had been abused before age 18 were at increased risk of having an unintended pregnancy. Among a sample of women considered to be at risk for acquiring HIV infection, those who reported sexual abuse were three times as likely as those who had not experienced abuse to become pregnant before 18 years of age. In a study of sexually experienced adolescents, those who had ever been forced to have sexual intercourse were significantly more likely than others to have ever been pregnant.

While it is clear that forced sexual intercourse may directly result in pregnancy among pubescent adolescents, the path by which sexual abuse at young ages leads to teenage pregnancy is less direct and requires exploration. Consideration of the nature and context of a girl's early sexual experiences is necessary in understanding why some teenagers may be more likely than others to become pregnant. Premature, exploitive and coercive sexual experiences may form the social-emotional context for early pregnancy. Among the possible consequences of childhood sexual abuse are promiscuity and the self-perception of being promiscuous; being the victim of coercive sex later in life; and poor self-concept, low self-esteem and decreased locus of control.

Girls may be placed at increased risk for early pregnancy if they fear that they are unable to conceive. In a study of low-income, nulliparous adolescents, those with a history of sexual abuse were more likely than others to report that they were trying to conceive and feared that they were unable to do so. Although the nature of sexual abuse reported in various studies may differ in terms of type, duration, and relationship and age of the victim and perpetrator, any unwanted sexual experience and the perception of abuse contribute to increased sexual risk behavior and low self-esteem.

In this study, we hypothesized that a history of perceived sexual abuse is associated with adolescent pregnancy and predisposes girls to early pregnancy because of early initiation of sexual activity and other sexual risk factors. Our study goes beyond previous research in this area by comparing the pregnancy experiences of girls who have been sexually abused with those of girls with no history of abuse.

Study Population and Instrument

We analyzed data from the Washington State Survey of Adolescent Health Behaviors, which was administered to a sample of sixth, eighth, 10th and 12th graders in 70 school districts in December 1992. The survey used a multiple-choice format, giving students up to five possible responses to questions about their ethnicity, drug and alcohol use, health risk factors, sexual activity, and experiences of physical and sexual abuse. Of the 120 questions, 14 asked about sexual activity, abuse and suicide. Some school districts and individual schools excluded this section from the questionnaire; where the questions were included, a preface indicated that students could choose not to answer them.

Surveys were distributed by teachers to each student in their class. Students were told their responses were anonymous and were instructed not to put their name on the response form and to seal their completed survey in an envelope. A designated student delivered all sealed envelopes to the school office.

Cluster sampling was used wherein schools were stratified by region, size and rurality in order to increase the chance of obtaining a representative sample of the Washington State school population. Schools were categorized as rural or urban using definitions from the 1990 census.

The initial sample consisted of 16,610 students. On the basis of quality control measures, 1,317 questionnaires were discarded because of apparently dishonest responses, out-of-range answers, impossible patterns or inconsistent responses. (For example, some girls responded that they had never had sexual intercourse, but also indicated that they had used birth control at last intercourse.) Also excluded were 10,833 questionnaires from males, sixth graders and girls whose school district did not include the questions about sexual activity, abuse and suicide, and 1,332 from girls whose school excluded these questions or who chose not to respond. The final sample included 3,128 girls in grades eight, 10 and 12.

Data and Analyses

The questionnaire asked respondents whether they had ever experienced sexual abuse (defined as "when someone in your family or someone else touches you in a sexual way in a place you did not want to be touched, or does something to you sexually which they shouldn't have done"), whether they had ever been "physically abused or mistreated by an adult," and the number of times they had been pregnant. It also asked about alcohol consumption (quantity and frequency) and drug use (types of drugs and frequency of use).

Teachers administering the survey recorded students' grade level on the questionnaires. The following variables, which we hypothesized would be linked with a report of sexual abuse, were measured by students' responses to multiple-choice survey questions: ethnicity; parental supervision (how often the respondent's parents knew her whereabouts); number of school activities and sports teams the respondent participated in; how frequently she missed school; importance of grades; current grades; plans to attend college; thoughts of dropping out of school; body image; sexual experience; age at first intercourse; number of sexual partners; birth control method used during last intercourse; and suicide thoughts, plans and attempts.

Because dichotomous variables are required for logistic regression analyses, responses to variables with a five-option response format were collapsed. For example, responses about drug use were collapsed into "no use" or "any use.". . .

Logistic regression techniques were used to measure differences between respondents who had been sexually abused and those who had not been abused. To test the hypothesis that sexual abuse contributes to early pregnancy via increased emphasis on sexuality and sexual risk-taking, a series of logistic regression analyses were performed to examine the degree to which a variety of factors were significant predictors of ever having had sexual intercourse and having been pregnant. . . .

Sexual Abuse

We found that sexual abuse was strongly associated with adolescent pregnancy, primarily through the strong association between sexual abuse and high-risk sexual behavior. The association between sexual abuse and adolescent pregnancy appears mediated in this way for two reasons. First, although a history of sexual abuse was strongly associated with reported sexual intercourse, it was not predictive of pregnancy among girls who had engaged in sexual intercourse. Second, when high-risk sexual behavior, which is strongly associated with sexual abuse, was added to a multivariate model, the effect of sexual abuse on pregnancy was no longer significant.

Clinicians and researchers who work with pregnant teenagers and adolescent parents have stressed that a better understanding of the social-emotional context of early sexual activity, especially premature or coercive sexual experiences, will contribute to understanding teenage pregnancy. Findings from this study suggest that premature and coercive sexual experiences contribute to adolescent pregnancy by increasing the likelihood that teenagers will have earlier sexual intercourse and a greater number of partners, and decreasing the likelihood that they will use birth control.

Among a sample of female students in grades 6–12, one study found that 18% had experienced an "unwanted" sexual encounter. Another analysis, in which sexual abuse was defined as unwanted sexual touching by an adult or by an older or stronger person either outside or inside the family, found a sexual abuse prevalence of 17% among a sample of school-based adolescent females. Similarly, in a sample of school-based adolescent females, the prevalence of forced sexual intercourse was 13%.

The prevalence of sexual abuse in our sample (23%) is higher than the rates reported for adolescents in different geographic regions, but is consistent with findings from retrospective studies that use a definition of sexual abuse not limited to forced sexual intercourse. The prevalence of sexual and physical abuse (60%) among ever-pregnant teenagers in this sample is similar to the prevalence documented for a sample of pregnant and parenting adolescents. The prevalence of sexual abuse among respondents who reported pregnancy (48%) is similar to that in other studies of pregnant adolescents.

Lack of Parental Supervision

The finding that respondents who reported sexual abuse were more likely than others to report a lack of parental supervision is supported by similar findings from an earlier epidemiological study. The overwhelming differences in negative social and health-related behaviors between the students who reported sexual abuse and those who did not expand upon findings from clinical or more limited samples and depict the sad accompaniments of sexual abuse.

Girls who either temporarily or permanently dropped out of school because of pregnancy were not included in the survey. Consequently, this sample represents only those who remained in or returned to school despite a pregnancy. It is possible that girls not in school at the time of the survey had different rates of sexual abuse and other risk factors from girls who remained in school.

Because this survey did not ask respondents the sequence in which pregnancy and abuse occurred, the abuse may have taken place after the pregnancy for some who reported both experiences. Biologically and developmentally, however, it seems more plausible that sexual victimization would have preceded pregnancy. Several epidemiologic studies have found that in the general population of women, 60–80% of incidents of abuse occur before 11 years of age, while

20–28% occur among adolescents. Studies of adolescent parents and pregnant teenagers have also reported young mean ages at first molestation (9.7 and 11.5 years, respectively).

We do not know whether this sample differs from other samples with regard to the age at onset of abuse or the proportion of girls abused during adolescence. In our sample, 18% of eighth graders and 28% of 12th graders reported a history of sexual abuse. This difference may reflect that as young girls age, they experience additional incidents of abuse, develop greater awareness of what constitutes abuse or become more willing to disclose prior abuse.

A small number of respondents may have become pregnant as a result of abuse. For them, at least one incident of abuse may have been directly related to a reported pregnancy.

Victims of Sexual Abuse

Studies of pregnant adolescents indicate a high rate of sexual victimization. Sexual abuse survivors are significantly more likely to become pregnant before age 18 than are their non-abused peers. Other surveys of pregnant or parenting teens found half to two-thirds reported sexual abuse histories.

Susan K. Flinn, *Advocates for Youth*, January 1995.

Further, because sexual abuse may be perpetrated by peers as well as older men, adolescent pregnancy may mask sexual abuse. Since the survey did not question respondents about the age of the perpetrator of sexual abuse, some may have reported on incidents involving peers. Consequently, findings must be interpreted according to a definition of sexual abuse that is not limited by the age of the perpetrator, but that encompasses any sexual experience perceived as forceful or coercive. However, in one analysis, the perpetrators of abuse were, on average, at least six years older than their victims, and many retrospective studies have indicated that perpetrators are at least five years older than their victims.

Some critics may question the authenticity of information regarding sexual abuse obtained via self-report. Cultural receptivity to reports of abuse has generally improved over time. Reasons for a girl not to report a history of sexual abuse far outweigh any speculations as to why one might falsely report sexual abuse on an anonymous survey. The tendency in reporting is to understate the prevalence of abuse. Further, the perception of abuse is equally important in predicting feelings of low self-esteem.

Physical Abuse and Early Pregnancy

Maltreatment of any kind has been increasingly implicated as a strong factor in adolescent pregnancy. The fact that pregnancy rates in this sample were also high among girls who suffered physical but not sexual abuse illustrates the need for further study of how a history of physical abuse contributes to an increased risk of early pregnancy. It is notable that in analyses controlling for grade level and sexual abuse, physical abuse approached significance as a factor predicting pregnancy and was significant in predicting the likelihood of ever having had sexual intercourse.

Also of importance is consideration of how nonparticipation in extracurricular activities could play a role in predicting pregnancy. Decreased participation may simply be a result of or concomitant with numerous predisposing risk factors. On the other hand, encouragement and support for girls to participate in activities may contribute to preventing early pregnancy.

Adolescent pregnancy is a multidimensional public health problem. Therefore, successful prevention strategies must address its many, complex aspects, including the important role of sexual abuse. Policy directives at the national level must set the stage for recognizing the costly consequences of sexual abuse. Thorough and routine inquiry regarding exposure to sexual abuse among school-age and adolescent girls may be helpful in targeting girls for prevention of teenage pregnancy, as well as for other needed counseling and support, particularly in the areas of sexual behavior and use of birth control.

Emphasis on primary prevention of undesirable experiences (for example, childhood and adolescent sexual abuse) would contribute to decreasing subsequent tragic and costly outcomes. The private nature of sexual abuse makes the task of primary prevention formidable, but crucial.

"Teenagers do not have problems because they have babies; they have babies because they have problems."

Poor Life Circumstances Contribute to Teenage Pregnancy

Richard T. Cooper

Efforts to reduce teenage pregnancy have led some people to consider the social and familial circumstances of adolescent mothers. Findings reflect an abundance of child abuse, poor parenting, and poverty in the lives of girls who have children as teenagers. In the following viewpoint, Richard T. Cooper describes the research of professor Joseph Hotz, who argues that deplorable life circumstances often result in pregnant teenagers. He claims that teen pregnancy is a symptom, rather than a cause, of the problems in girls' lives. Cooper is a staff writer for the *Los Angeles Times*.

As you read, consider the following questions:
1. Why, according to Hotz, is there little difference between girls who have babies in their teens and similar girls who wait until their twenties, as quoted by the author?
2. What are three similarities the author describes between Aurora Lopez and Khadija Robinson?
3. According to the author, what benefits might a young woman perceive in having a child in her teens?

In May 1997, with a fanfare of support from the White House and Capitol Hill, a coalition of liberals and conservatives called the National Campaign to Prevent Teen Pregnancy launched a . . . crusade. Its goals: To increase awareness of the devastating problems faced by adolescent mothers and to cut the teen pregnancy rate one-third by the year 2005.

Americans, the group declared, "see teen pregnancy as a powerful marker of a society gone astray—a clear and compelling example of how our families, communities and common culture are under siege." Experts warned of the link between teenage childbearing and multigenerational poverty, crime, joblessness and high welfare costs.

Then First Lady Hillary Rodham Clinton hosted a reception. MTV pledged to develop public service announcements. Scriptwriters and producers for ABC's daytime television shows offered to help. Black Entertainment Television and the hip hop/rap group Salt-N-Pepa lent a hand.

So serious is the problem in California, which has the highest teen pregnancy rate of any state, that then Governor Pete Wilson . . . launched a massive advertising blitz in 1996 warning teens against the burdens of childbearing. . . .

Somehow, though, when the campaign against teen pregnancy was kicking off in Washington, V. Joseph Hotz's invitation must have been lost in the mail.

That can happen if you're the sort of person who tries to sell sour apples to Betty Crocker. And when it comes to teenage childbearing, Hotz is a sour-apples kind of guy.

An economist and social policy specialist with a PhD from the University of Wisconsin, 11 years on the faculty of the University of Chicago and a . . . faculty appointment at UCLA, Hotz is the very model of a modern professional scholar. He was commissioned by a foundation fighting teen pregnancy to mount a major study of the issue.

But he came to conclusions that many in the fight against teen pregnancy and childbearing now wish would simply go away.

Hotz has found that being a teenager has almost nothing to do with the problems that afflict most such females and their children. Teenage childbearing is a symptom, he says, not a cause. Teenagers do not have problems because they have babies; they have babies because they have problems.

Even if they had put off having children for a few years—until they were no longer teenagers—it would make little difference, Hotz contends. They would still be grindingly poor, still collect welfare, still have terrible jobs and difficult lives. So would their children.

The problems they suffer from are so severe and began so early in their lives that it makes little difference whether they have babies as teenagers or a few years later. Focusing on their age diverts attention from the real causes of their problems, he says, and makes solutions harder to achieve. . . .

Different Women, Similar Lives

According to the conventional view, Aurora Lopez has done it right. In her mid-20s, she is only now expecting her first baby. She finished high school in her native Nicaragua and even attended college there for a time.

Khadija Robinson, by contrast, had her first child when she was 15. She dropped out of school in junior high, had three more children by two fathers—all out of wedlock—and now depends on welfare, food stamps and the generosity of the grandmother of three of her children.

Lopez and Robinson seem to represent, on the one hand, how things should be, and, on the other, all that is disturbing about teen pregnancy. In reality, however, the lives of the two women are strikingly similar; so are their bleak prospects.

Together, they lend support to the view that a complex web of factors determines who is likely to become a young, unwed mother—factors that begin early in life and cast their shadow well beyond the teen years. Both Lopez and Robinson, who asked that their real names not be used, are the daughters of teenage, single mothers who had little education and bore many children. Both grew up in extreme poverty without fathers at home.

Lopez was severely beaten and abused by her mother. Robinson and one of her brothers were taken away from their mother by authorities after the children were left alone and the little boy was scalded in a kitchen accident. Robinson was repeatedly beaten by the grandmother who took her in.

Today, neither Lopez nor Robinson has many skills to offer the job market. Lopez, who speaks limited English, has found only part-time work, in a neighborhood grocery store that pays her $140—cash, no benefits—for three long days' work each week. She shares a one-bedroom apartment with her father, a hotel kitchen worker, and her brother, her sister and her sister's three children.

Robinson, now 20, has too many children to work. Thanks to classes at a teen parent center, however, she expects to have earned a general equivalency diploma by the end of this year; she's good at math and dreams of more schooling and a bookkeeping job.

Both Lopez and Robinson face their lives with nearly equal parts apprehension and luminous hope. "I will need to be more responsible than before because I have to take care of another person's life—be the mama," says Lopez. "And it's for life."

"It will be hard," Robinson agrees. "I've got a long way to go. I try my best to make it as easy as possible, but it's going to be hard because I'm struggling now."

What makes it worth the struggle, she declares, is her children. "They're the best thing in my life. They'll always be there, when everybody else turns their back on you."

Not the First to Question Cause

Grandson of an Irish immigrant housekeeper for the parish priest, husband of a seventh-grade math teacher, father of two children, Joe Hotz is as mainstream as they come. He is not even the first to question the idea that having a baby as a teenager causes the manifold problems that follow.

Arline T. Geronimus of the University of Michigan and Sanders Korenman of the National Bureau of Economic Research had already conducted studies casting doubt on teenage childbearing as the cause of later problems. Ethnographic studies by Elijah Anderson of the University of Pennsylvania, who has explored the sociological roots of the problem, pointed to similar conclusions.

Hotz's breakthrough was to develop a method for comparing teenage mothers with a group of their peers—a formidable task because, even in the poor, minority neighborhoods in which most teen mothers live, they are significantly more disadvantaged than most other young women around them.

Hotz and his colleagues, using data from a study that has been following a large group of young women for many years, extracted a sample of who had had babies as teenagers and another group who had become pregnant as teens but had lost their babies to miscarriages and had children only later.

Community Effort

Helping our communities prevent teen pregnancy is an important mission. Unmarried teenagers who become pregnant face severe emotional, physical, and financial difficulties. The children born to unmarried teenagers will struggle to fulfill the promise given to all human life, and many of them simply will not succeed. Many of them will remain trapped in a cycle of poverty, and unfortunately may become part of our criminal justice system.

Michael N. Castle, "Statement on National Teen Pregnancy Prevention Month," May 12, 1999.

When Hotz's team looked at how the lives of the two sets of women had turned out, some startling conclusions emerged:
- By their mid-30s, the teen mothers had worked harder and longer and earned more money than their counterparts who had their first babies later. Both groups had collected welfare, but the teen mothers had paid more taxes and on balance cost taxpayers less.
- The teen mothers got about as much education as their peers who deferred childbearing. Fewer graduated from high school, but more got GEDs.
- Problems of alcohol and drug abuse were no more common among the teen mothers than among the other group.

Even the children of teenage mothers may not do significantly worse than the offspring of similarly disadvantaged but somewhat older peers, Hotz thinks, though this point remains disputed.

What explains these findings?

First, the problems afflicting teen mothers are generally so serious that the passage of a few years does little to erase them.

Second, most teenage mothers belong to communities in which having children at a relatively early age is the norm. The practical question is not whether prospective teen mothers can be induced to wait as long as middle-class women do; the question is whether they can be persuaded to wait until their early 20s, and whether doing so would make much difference—especially since two-thirds of all teen mothers are 18 or 19 years old when they have their first babies.

Third, since poor, severely disadvantaged women must compete near the bottom of the labor market, where credentials are less important than steady performance, there may be benefits to getting childbearing out of the way early, when earnings potential is lowest, and then beginning an uninterrupted work career.

Findings Upset Issue's Politics

When all is said and done, what makes Joe Hotz as unwelcome as mold on bread is not so much his research as the politics of the issue.

Teenage pregnancy, childbearing and unwed motherhood are difficult issues at best. But they have become a battleground in the ideological struggle between Left and Right. Hotz's findings are awkward for all concerned.

He offers little support for conservatives who would cast the issue in terms of personal morality and who advocate stern measures against unwed mothers.

His research is also picklish for traditional liberal advocacy groups. The message that teen mothers do no worse than others calls into question the wisdom of focusing so heavily on adolescents, as many socially conscious liberals have been doing. His analysis could also be used to justify less government effort.

Even moderates find little reason to trumpet Hotz's work. The National Campaign to Prevent Teen Pregnancy, for example, is laboring to find ways to sidestep the ideological conflicts and find practical strategies both sides can accept. Giving the spotlight to Hotz's work could stir controversy and make it harder to build such coalitions. At the same time, the campaign wants to encourage better research on the issue.

So campaign officials, reflecting the dilemma of those in the middle, don't challenge Hotz's findings but they don't go out of their way to trumpet them either. Kristen Moore, a campaign board member and respected researcher in the field, agrees with the thrust of Hotz's work.

"The kids who become teen parents in a modern industrial society are not average kids," Moore says. "The kids who have births are actually disadvantaged across a wide array of background characteristics. And so it's not surprising that they are doing poorly. They would have been doing poorly anyhow."

But she and others are quick to add that teen childbearing rates are far higher in the United States than in other advanced countries and insist that they can and should be brought down.

Baby Gives Her Mother Inspiration

Meanwhile, a few blocks from the Capitol and half a light-year away from the policy wars, 18-year old Miriam Turcios and her 15-month old daughter go about the business of keeping on keeping on.

Turcios receives government assistance and, with help from the "Healthy Families" program at Mary's Center, a city-supported center for young mothers, she worked throughout her pregnancy, is about to graduate from high school and has even applied to college.

"The baby inspired me to do a lot more than I did before," she says. "That's the reason she's here, I guess, to inspire me. Things are difficult right now, but I'm striving to do better. I'm stronger than I was before.

"My route has a lot of bumps in it, but I'll get there."

5

> *"Do [myths about sex] originate with misinformed parents or is the only knowledge teens obtain about sexuality through even less-informed peers?"*

A Lack of Accurate Sex Information Contributes to Teenage Pregnancy

Jo Ann Wentzel

With so many different sex education programs, public service announcements, and television programs, it is difficult to believe that some teenagers do not have all the facts about sex and its possible consequences. In the following viewpoint, senior editor Jo Ann Wentzel describes some of the myths surrounding sexuality that teenagers have told her. She argues that unless teenagers are taught about sex, pregnancy, and sexually transmitted infections, they will continue to have unprotected sex and make babies before they are ready for the responsibility of parenthood. Wentzel is affiliated with *Parenting Today's Teen*, an online publication dedicated to fostering better communication and relationships between teenagers and parents.

As you read, consider the following questions:

1. What are two myths about pregnancy told to Wentzel?
2. What are three reasons Wentzel offers for why girls allow themselves to get pregnant as teenagers?
3. What advice does Wentzel offer teenagers as the best way to avoid pregnancy?

"We know what causes that now," I said, smiling at her. "Huh?" she replied in her usually perceptive way.

I pointed to her rather stretched pregnant tummy attached to her 16-year-old body.

"Oh, that's not very funny."

"No, pregnancy isn't," I agreed. "Especially when you're not yet grown yourself."

This conversation with teenage girls has taken place way too many times. . . . *Parenting Today's Teen* contracted with counties to put independent teens into their own apartments. This was just one of the many girls we served in our program, Life Ready. Half the girls we worked with were pregnant before we started, some after, but all very pregnant. I was saddened as I sat across from another teenager who had lost her childhood and would bring another unfortunate baby into the world unwanted or at least unprepared for by these teens.

Talking with dozens of young ladies who are soon-to-be moms, I questioned them about how—with all the information and free contraception devices available—they had become pregnant.

The answers I heard are as amazing as they are stupid, but these myths still exist among our teens. Hopefully, this will encourage [everyone] to educate teens . . . about the realities of sex and one of its consequences—pregnancy.

Pregnancy Myths

I was told by one young lady she just could not believe she was pregnant.

"Did you not have intercourse with a young man?" I questioned.

"Yes," she replied.

"Well, did you use any kind of contraceptive?" further seeking an explanation for her bewilderment.

"No," she admitted.

"Then why are you surprised you are pregnant?"

"Because it was my very first time, and everyone knows you can't get pregnant your first time."

Sadly, I had heard this same myth before. Where do teens get these ideas? Do they originate with misinformed parents or is the only knowledge teens obtain about sexuality through even less-informed peers? Is this a line young boys use when everything else fails? Do these young girls actually believe those lines?

Another "favorite" myth of mine was revealed by a young woman practicing labor breathing and effleurage. She satisfied every question about why she was in her present condition when she said, "But I was not even undressed all the way." I waited for further explanation, but that was it.

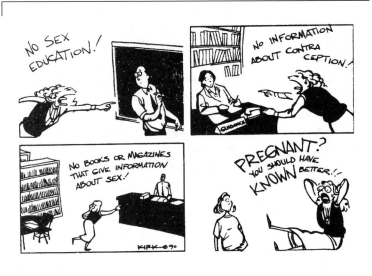

Kirk. © 1990 by Kirk Anderson. Reprinted with permission.

Apparently, if you wear a few clothing items while engaging in intercourse, you will be safe. Great news! Where do you purchase this contraceptive clothing?

Did you know that if you spend the night instead of having a quick romp in a back seat, you can't get pregnant? I have that explanation on "good authority." So forget curfew, because if you stay until morning, no baby will be on the way.

Where does this misinformation come from, and why do these kids believe it? Isn't sex-ed taught to clear up these types of myths? Why haven't the parents cleared this up? My guess is that this is one area parents still don't talk about. A common parental myth is if you don't want your kids to engage in sex, don't talk about it. Here's a news flash, they already are having sex! Give them the blasted facts!

Then we have the "I didn't use a condom because he said he can't feel anything with one on. Or "Jeff says it isn't real that way."

We also have the sad commentary on why girls let this happen. First, there's the everyone's-having-sex-you-gotta-do-it-to-be-cool syndrome. Then there's the "we really love each other and I wanted to show him" routine. But saddest of all is when a girl told me she wanted something of her own that she could love. "I needed someone to love me no matter what." Our teens are searching for unconditional love that their families haven't given them. They are hoping this tiny infant fills their needs, when it should be the baby getting his or her needs met.

They want love and they confuse it with sex. When sex brings about a small life, they feel they have found love. They are so busy getting love, they may not ever learn how to give it. And so the cycle continues, and another child is born who does not have its needs met.

A Plea to Teens

Teenagers, please wait to have babies. My advice is to abstain from sex, but you won't listen, so at least have protected sex. Babies should be born out of love because they are wanted. They should be welcomed and anxiously awaited. They should not be the result of a union taking place between two kids who don't even know each other's name.

The reasons to not have babies are numerous. First, you need time to grow up, and your childhood is extinguished as soon as you are pregnant. The health and safety reasons for not having sex you probably know, but ignore. Pregnancy, AIDS and venereal disease are real possibilities. Yes, it can happen to you!

Your education will be shortened and your options will be lessened if you become pregnant while very young. Programs exist, but are difficult to get into. Your chances of keeping the baby, school and a job going—and having a social life—are almost nonexistent.

Learn the facts about sex, contraceptives and pregnancy.

Make good choices. Don't have sex just to have something to do. It may be an activity to your group just like going to the movies or going roller blading, but the consequences can be deadly.

It's easy to protect yourself from pregnancy, the grounding that lasts 18 years, because we know what causes that now.

Periodical Bibliography

The following articles have been selected to supplement the diverse views presented in this chapter.

Donna Britt	"For Every Single Mom, a Singular Life Story," *Washington Post*, June 22, 2001.
Jane D. Brown and Sarah N. Keller	"Can the Mass Media Be Healthy Sex Educators?" *Family Planning Perspectives*, September/October 2000.
Catherine Elton	"Jail Baiting: Statutory Rape's Dubious Comeback," *New Republic*, October 20, 1997.
Kevin Fiscella et al.	"Does Child Abuse Predict Adolescent Pregnancy?" *Pediatrics*, April 1998.
Jewel L. Jones Harris	"Urban African American Adolescent Parents: Their Perspectives of Sex, Love, Intimacy, Pregnancy, and Parenting," *Adolescence*, Winter 1998.
Ariel Kalil and Sandra K. Danziger	"How Teen Mothers Are Faring Under Welfare Reform," *Journal of Social Issues*, Winter 2000.
Michael W. Lynch	"Enforcing Statutory Rape?" *Public Interest*, July 15, 1998.
Mona McCullough and Avraham Scherman	"Family-of-Origin Interaction and Adolescent Mothers' Potential for Child Abuse," *Adolescence*, Summer 1998.
Elizabeth Mehren	"Statutory Rape: When Is a Crime Not a Crime?" *Los Angeles Times*, August 6, 1997.
David Popenoe	"Teen Pregnancy: An American Dilemma," Testimony before the House of Representatives, Committee on Small Business, Subcommittee on Empowerment, Washington, DC, July 16, 1998.
K. Lynne Robinson et al.	"Rural Junior High School Students' Risk Factors for and Perceptions of Teenage Parenthood," *Journal of School Health*, October 1998.
Christine Siegworth Meyer and Swati Mukerjee	"Black Teen Childbearing: Reexamining the Segmented Labor Market Hypothesis," *Review of Black Political Economy*, Spring 2000.
Janet I. Tu	"A Family Tradition She'd Like to End: Teen Pregnancy," *Seattle Times*, January 23, 2000.

CHAPTER 3

What Options Are Available to Pregnant Teenagers?

Chapter Preface

Every year, about 40 percent of teenage girls who become pregnant in the United States choose to have an abortion. Around 274,000 abortions were performed on teenage girls in 1996. This figure has caused much controversy between people who advocate a teenager's right to choose abortion and those who argue in favor of her unborn child.

Pro-life advocates argue that a young girl should not be able to have an abortion, because it violates an unborn child's right to life. They contend that abortion is murder and is therefore unethical. According to the Teachers for Life Association, "Abortion kills an unborn child. A society that allows abortion is denying the most fundamental human right—the right to life—to one group of human beings, the unborn." Although some abortion critics make exceptions for teenagers whose pregnancies result from rape or incest, others maintain that the unborn baby should not have to pay for the criminal act of its father. Many abortion opponents argue that the child's basic right to life overrides any other considerations, including the mother's welfare.

However, supporters of abortion maintain that a woman should have the right to decide what to do with her body and when to become a parent. Moreover, they argue that most teenage pregnancies are unplanned, and most teenage girls are too immature to become parents. Abortion rights activists claim that it is immoral to force the responsibility of raising a child on someone who is not ready for parenthood. As stated by Diana Alstad of the National Abortion Rights Action League, "Choosing abortion to avoid having an unwanted child should be looked upon as a moral act, instead of a regrettable one. Bringing a child into the world that cannot be adequately cared for is what should be seen as truly regrettable. I view forcing any woman, no matter what her age, to have a child that she doesn't want or is unprepared to raise, as a totally immoral act in this day and age."

Statistics reveal that teenage abortions declined by about 31 percent during the period between 1986 and 1996. The authors in the following chapter debate what the best option is for a teenager who is faced with an unplanned pregnancy.

| "*I'm coming to terms with the concept that my decision [to have an abortion] was not only best for me, but best for the child.*"

Abortion Is an Option for Pregnant Teenagers

Elisabeth Pruden

In the following viewpoint, Elisabeth Pruden argues that abortion is sometimes the best solution for pregnant teenagers. Describing her own decision to have an abortion as a teenager, she claims that she, like many other young girls, did not have enough support from either her family or the father of her baby to raise a child. Moreover, carrying the baby to term and giving it up for adoption was an undesirable option because of the social stigma attached to unwed pregnancy and the uncertainty of the baby's future. Pruden, who is now married with one child, maintains that although her decision to abort her baby was difficult, it enabled her to finish her education and later—when she was ready for it—start a family.

As you read, consider the following questions:
1. According to Pruden, how do people react when she reveals that she had an abortion?
2. How did the author's boyfriend react when she told him she was pregnant?
3. Why does Pruden claim that she would not be married to her husband if she had not had the abortion as a teenager?

Nothing changes someone's opinion of you quicker than revealing to them you've had an abortion. Some people are genuinely curious about your experience, and respect your right to control your own body as well as your own destiny.

Others (and in my experience these "others" constitute the majority), tense up and recoil from you, as if you'd just informed them you are carrying the Ebola virus and are highly contagious. As someone who has never had an impenetrable shield of high self-esteem, it's been difficult to get used to.

Keeping Secrets

Not that I'm just running around telling every person I come across about my dirty little secret. For a long, long time I told no one, including the wonderful saint of a guy I'm now married to. But, as my mind processed the emotional aftermath of the abortion, I realized it was something I shouldn't have to carry around inside of me like a big, black spot on my otherwise healthy soul. That epiphany led to the next logical conclusion—if I was having trouble coming to terms with what that event meant for me as a person and what it meant for my future, other young women were probably grappling with the same thing. Maybe by becoming active and sharing my experiences, I could help someone else deal with what I had had to confront alone.

Whenever I see a blurb on the news about the abortion controversy, my interest is piqued, as if big, flashing neon arrows are pointing to the television. Never mind if the stock market just fell through the floor or if every nation in the world just declared war on the United States—here's something that actually relates directly to my life for a change. My point of view is rather unique because I've been on both sides of the fence when it comes to abortion, so to speak. As a young teenager, I had an abortion; a few years later I was pregnant again, but this time I chose to carry the baby to term and raise her. And last summer, I miscarried my third pregnancy.

Each one of those pregnancies rocked the foundations of my self-concept and tinted my view of the world and what is important in it. It still amazes me that an ancient, primitive biological process—reproduction—has the power to change the center of my own personal universe and arouse such passion in people with differing viewpoints and experiences.

My Conservative Hometown

Before my first pregnancy, I considered myself decidedly pro-choice, and I still do, although my reasons have changed. My hometown has a reputation for its conservative, religious-right attitudes (hell, it's President George W. Bush's hometown), and many houses had signs in the front yard with the oh-so-catchy little slogan, "It's a baby, y'all."

In the throes of my rebellious teenage angst, the signs drove me completely nuts. Late at night, after the town had rolled up the sidewalks and all the good boys and girls were safely in bed, my high school girlfriends and I would dress in black and make drive-by alterations to these nifty little signs.

I'd dash out of the car and race to the sign in the unsuspecting victim's yard, and with my jumbo, industrial-strength black permanent marker, obliterate the word 'baby' and write in 'choice' so that the new and improved version now proclaimed, "It's a choice, y'all."

What righteous rebels we were then. However, at that point, my enthusiasm for choice was purely intellectual. I had never been pregnant, or even known anyone my age who had been. Life at that point centered around prom and clothes and getting through the next band practice.

The deep emotional turmoil of facing an unplanned pregnancy was unfathomable to me and I was just not mature enough to realize that some things are more important than having an acceptable date to Homecoming. Beliefs I thought I had weren't really convictions until they were tested by fire. And shortly after those carefree, independent days, the fates would indeed see what I was made of.

My Baby's Father

I met Ryan through a friend of a friend just as school was starting in September. I immediately found myself disliking him. He was older, he was brilliantly smart and he was quite the hottie to boot. Sounds perfect, right? The problem was, he knew all that, and had the ego to go along with it. For weeks I could barely stand being in his presence, and only endured him because my best friend had decided he should be the newest member of our clique.

By Thanksgiving, I had broken up with my longtime boyfriend and found myself single again. I had been the type of girl who always had a boyfriend, and I didn't know what to do with myself. So, when Ryan asked me out, I agreed.

As we became closer, I came to see that he was even more flawed emotionally than I had previously thought, but we had an incredible, almost surreal, chemistry and I realized we viewed the world in much the same way. Eventually it was those flaws that drew me to him and blinded me to what would be the inevitable result of our lustful relationship. I was in love, and it was bad.

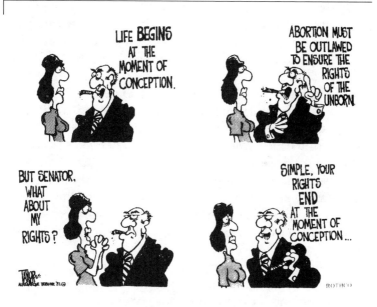

Taylor. © 1982 by Taylor/Rothco. Reprinted with permission.

In late December, just after Christmas, I realized my period hadn't come like it should have. Immediately, I filled with panic and raced to Wal-Mart for a pregnancy test. My hands were shaking uncontrollably as I watched the dreaded second line appear in the little window. My heart was pounding so hard I thought I would pass out. What the hell was I going to do? As much as my heart wanted Ryan to take me in his arms and say, "That's wonderful news, let's get married and have this baby," I knew it wouldn't happen.

We were so young, and Ryan had grand dreams of entering politics and changing the world. As he so sensitively put it, "I can't be President of the United States and have some illegitimate kid running around somewhere."

My friends were supportive, and eventually Ryan lost the respect of everyone in our group, and left town. Last I heard he was wandering around Canada somewhere.

Making Decisions

Naturally, I was in denial for a while. There was no way in hell I could keep this baby, I thought. My mom was definitely not the type to give unconditional love and support to her pregnant teenage daughter; my dad was pretty much estranged from us and was the last person I thought of going to for help. Never in my young life had I felt so completely alone and doomed.

But gradually, through the love of some great friends, I began to see the situation from a larger perspective. It wasn't just me whose life was going to be profoundly affected, there was this tiny little embryo in there that depended completely on me. Adoption was not something I considered, because going through with the pregnancy would, without a doubt, get me disowned and thrown out on the street. Plus, I knew I would never be able to go on with my life always wondering where my baby was, and if she were being loved, and not abused.

My options, as they appeared to me that cold, gray winter, were to either keep the child and live completely on my own, young and with no education, with no means of providing any kind of appropriate life for my child, or have an abortion. Ultimately, the choice was clear, but it still broke my heart.

Since then, I've developed into a more mature, altruistic, and confident person. Because of that experience, I realized the importance of getting a good education and thus the means of providing for a family. A few years later, while at college, I received a letter from my first high school sweetheart. We hadn't talked in about two years, and even though I had moved on with my life and become somewhat self-sufficient, I always knew we'd end up together.

A New Baby

Soon we were engaged, and a few months after that I was pregnant again. What a world of difference it made having the right guy beside me this time. Although we were still young, and not yet finished with college, the thought of having an abortion never crossed either of our minds; we knew we were in it for the long haul.

On St. Patrick's Day in 1999, our daughter came sliding into the world, screaming and making her substantial presence known. She has taught me much about abortion and the older sibling she never had, and with every milestone she reached in her first year, I wondered what would have been had my circumstances and decisions been different a few years earlier.

I know that I would not have my daughter or my husband today if I had kept the first baby; my husband would have assumed that having a child by another guy meant there was no place for him in my life, and thus we wouldn't be together now. And I can't imagine my life without my beautiful, strong-willed, two-year-old baby.

Personal Choices

My abortion has been called a selfish decision by some, and others have gone so far as to condemn me to burn in hell. But I figure that if there is indeed a hell and that's where I end up spending eternity, it will be for reasons other than having an abortion. I'm coming to terms with the concept that my decision was not only best for me, but best for the child who would have suffered a harsh and poverty-stricken life with no family to lovingly buffer the cruel realities of daily life.

Call me what you will, but before you condemn a young woman for choosing abortion, take a long, hard look at your own motives. Hopefully you'll realize that it is much easier to tell someone what they should do when you're not in their shoes. And when you decide that you are free from sin, let me be the first to congratulate you.

But women facing unplanned pregnancies don't need to be made to feel like murderers for choosing abortion, they need to be educated about the consequences of any decision they may make, and, most importantly, receive non-judgmental support from friends, family, and society.

> "Not only am I a product of a teenage, unplanned pregnancy, but I am also a female that believes she should not have the abortion option."

Abortion Should Not Be an Option for Pregnant Teenagers

Liz Kleemeier

In the following viewpoint, student Liz Kleemeier argues that abortion should not be an option for pregnant teenagers. As the product of an unplanned teenage pregnancy—she was adopted at birth—she contends that the life of an unborn child is well worth the hardship that a teenage mother faces. She maintains that more pregnant teenagers should consider putting their babies up for adoption, rather than having an abortion. Kleemeier is a student at the University of Dayton in Ohio.

As you read, consider the following questions:
1. What are two of the arguments the author suggests abortion rights advocates offer to protect the legality of abortion?
2. Why does the author claim that rape and incest are not sufficient reasons to abort one's child?
3. Why, according to Kleemeier, is pro-life "pro-woman"?

From "'Unwanted' Pregnancy Produces Pro-Choice's Worst Nightmare," by Liz Kleemeier, www.sjnews.org, August 13, 2001. Copyright © 2000 by Liz Kleemeier. Reprinted with permission.

My name is Liz Kleemeier, and I am proof that abortion is not necessary, a living example of how to handle a problem pregnancy without killing the baby. A woman like me is the abortion industry's worst enemy. Not only am I a product of a teenage, unplanned pregnancy, but I am also a female that believes she should not have the abortion option.

Abortion advocates offer many arguments for protecting the legality of abortion in this country. Some arguments include "How can I, a man, ever attempt to understand the circumstances surrounding a woman's right to choose?" Or, "we . . . are in no position to judge." There is the example of rape, saying that a woman not given the abortion, HAD she become pregnant, would be given a life long reminder of a heinous crime. Some say they know abortion is wrong, but view it as "not their business, so deal with it and move on."

To that I say, "my life IS my business," and I resent the abortion laws of this country telling me otherwise.

Years ago a teenager became pregnant and knew that my life was worth any difficulty a teenage pregnancy would entail. She knew I was alive within her, and she let my heart beat on, strong and steady, proclaiming life. She is my hero, and I am thankful.

Abortion Should Not Be Taken Lightly

Abortion has become a form of birth control in this country. A female director of a New York abortion clinic was asked why women have abortions. She said she is "sick and tired of hearing women don't do this lightly." Of her own clinic, she said, "Ninety-eight percent of women do it lightly in here . . . They think of abortion like brushing their . . . teeth, and that's okay with me." According to abortionists themselves approximately 95% of abortions are performed for social problems. The other 5% involves birth defects, health threat to mother, and rape and incest.

In defense of babies with birth defects, a young woman in Cincinnati recently became pregnant and wanted to give her baby up for adoption. Tests showed that the baby had Down Syndrome, and the Cincinnati Right to Life found a waiting list of 30 couples in the Cincinnati area waiting to adopt Down Syndrome babies. Life is truly beautiful in all forms, and God calls us to respect it.

In cases of health threat to the mother, I stand by the Catholic teaching: if a baby dies as a result of trying to save a mother's life, then the death of the baby is not murder.

Finally, in cases of rape and incest, murdering the baby serves to execute capital punishment for the crime of the father. A child should never have to pay with their life for the crime of another. In these cases the woman already has the lifelong reminder of a rape or incest. I know girls who have been raped and I doubt they will forget the crime any sooner than a woman who has become pregnant through rape. Abortions in these cases add to the trauma, as the woman will later remember the rape and abortion.

Women Choosing Life

I ask you to consider a survey that speaks for itself. Planned Parenthood, the largest abortion provider in the country, conducted a survey of women who had had abortions. Of the women, 39,000 had joined the National Abortion Rights Action League, the largest pro-abortion organization in the country. 245,000 of the polled women had joined the National Right to Life Committee, the largest pro-life organization in the country. Apparently, women who have had abortions are more likely to oppose abortion than to defend it. Pro-life IS pro-woman, as it fights to keep women from falling into the clutches of the abortion industry.

I would like to share my thoughts on one of the most often used arguments of the abortion industry: "It is none of your business, you are going to have to deal with it and move on." If you see someone being beaten on the street, is it right to just keep walking and justify it by saying "the attacker will just deal with God someday"? No. If someone knew that Susan Smith [who was convicted of two counts of murder in 1995] was planning to drown her sons, would abortion advocates condemn him for interfering? Susan has said that in her despair, it seemed to be her only choice.

It was a terrible and difficult decision. What would have given anyone the right to interfere in the most difficult decision Susan ever made? Susan probably would be grateful today if someone had interfered. During the Jewish Holocaust, should the United States have stood back and let Hitler go about his business, saying "God will let him know it's wrong eventually"? No. The question is not "what right do we have to interfere?" It is "what right do we have to abandon these women just when they need us most?" That is a question rarely asked, and almost never answered.

National Teens for Life

More than 30 million children have been killed since the U.S. Supreme Court legalized abortion in 1973. They were our brothers, sisters, cousins, nieces and nephews. They could have been anyone and anything. They would have been our friends. It is in their memory that we work to put an end to abortion. . . .

Our parents' generation gave us *Roe vs. Wade* and legalized abortion-on-demand. It is up to us to reverse our country's trend toward death and destruction. By working together we can, and will, restore a basic respect for life in America, as well as the world.

National Teens for Life, www.nrlc.org.

Now we face the American Holocaust against those who cannot protect themselves, as abortion targets the most innocent of our society. We will all be judged someday, and God will call for an accounting of our lives. However, God will not judge us solely on our sinful actions, but also for our lack of taking a stand against the evil in this world. It is too easy to look the other way in this world of convenience.

Consider Adoption

There are millions of couples in the United States on waiting lists to adopt these "unplanned" babies. Planned Parenthood uses the slogan "Every child a wanted child." By Planned Parenthood's standards, as a teenage pregnancy, I was not a wanted child. Tell that to my parents, who spent five years on a waiting list to carry me home from the adoption agency, and another four years to get my brother. I thank God for the patience of my parents, who have embedded me with strong Catholic faith and values by their example. When the adoption agency phoned them and said "we have a baby girl, do you want her?" they said yes and so I was born into the Kleemeier family.

My mother is always there to console me with a gentle touch and kind words when I am frustrated by the pro-abortion world around me. The biological mothers of my brother and I allowed God to guide us into the welcoming arms of the wonderful person I call "mom." My father spends each Saturday morning, rain, shine, or snow, picketing abortion clinics. God's will burns in his heart as he prays and endures being spat upon, screamed at, and hated for reaching out in love to strangers, only a rosary and prayers as his defense. His eyes have seen woman after woman drive up in everything from the cheapest to the most expensive cars, enter the clinic, have her money taken, her baby killed, and shoved into the parking lot to bleed. I remember my family standing together during the Life Chains of years past, hand in hand. God's hands made us a family and a beautiful one at that.

I hope that today I have been able to offer a different perspective on abortion, adoption, and what "right to life" really means. I have made fighting abortion my business. I will stand up to the pro-abortionists and let the fruits of my life serve as proof that unplanned pregnancies can have awesome results. Abortion should not be an option: My life is the most priceless gift anyone has ever given me. I believe it was a beautiful choice.

> *"I knew, without a doubt in my mind, that [giving up my baby for adoption] was the right decision to make."*

Adoption Is an Option for Pregnant Teenagers

Rebecca Lanning

Although most teenagers do not consider adoption a solution to teen pregnancy, some girls find it a good option. In the following viewpoint, Rebecca Lanning relates the story of Amy, a young girl who gave up her child for adoption. Amy maintains that adoption was the best decision for her and her child because her son's adoptive family was better able to provide economic and familial stability than she was. Rebecca Lanning is a contributor to *Teen Magazine*.

As you read, consider the following questions:
1. Why did Amy move out of her parents' house?
2. From what did Amy draw the most comfort at the Gladney Center?
3. Why did Amy feel awkward going back to public school?

At first, Amy felt as if her whole life was over. She cried a lot and agonized over how she could've avoided the situation. She wished that it was all just a bad dream. But as time passed, reality set in and suddenly she was faced with one of the toughest decisions of her life. Here, in her own words, she describes what happened when she found out she was pregnant and what she decided to do about it.

Amy's Story

"When I was 15, almost 16, Eric and I started dating. He was a year older than me, and I really felt like I was in love with him, but my parents absolutely hated him from the moment we started going out. He was a wild one, and I was just an innocent little girl. I had always lived a pretty sheltered life. I was attracted to Eric because he was wild and crazy, and I was totally different from him. We lied to my parents all the time and went out together.

About three months into the relationship, he started mentioning sex just to get my opinion on it. I was curious about it to say the least. It was never something that I could discuss with my parents. It was always, 'Don't do it,' and that was it. He mentioned it now and then, and he promised that I wouldn't get pregnant, nothing would happen, my parents would never have to know. And so we did have sex. He was my first, but I was not his. He'd been with a lot of girls. I was so immature. I had no idea what I was doing and what risks were involved. He told me everything would be OK, but in March, about a month after we started having sex, I was pregnant.

Taking the Test

When my period was late, I took an at-home pregnancy test. Eric was there with me. When we found out it was positive, I absolutely died. I pretty much knew it deep in my heart, but when we saw the results we just sat there and cried. We were both really scared. I had told my mom I was late, and she asked the next week if I had started and I told her no. She said, 'Well, could you be pregnant?' and I said, 'Yes.' She just started crying. My dad wouldn't even look at me, or he would look at me and shake his head. For three days, he didn't talk to me. When he finally did say something, it was, 'I hope you're happy. You've screwed up your entire life.' They were extremely disappointed.

I didn't know what to do. At first, Eric and I seriously talked about getting married, getting an apartment, having the perfect, fairy-tale life. I did some checking as to how much it was going to cost in terms of daycare and an apartment. We were both in high school. Neither of us had jobs; we both lived with our parents. Eventually, I realized there was just no way. At that point, when I realized the full extent of the situation, I considered abortion, but only for a minute. I knew that that just wasn't something I could do.

While all this was going on, I ended up leaving home. My parents and I were having such a hard time getting along. I felt so condemned by them. They couldn't believe I had gone against what they had tried to teach me. My mom kept saying, 'I can't believe you gave yourself to Eric!' She reminded me of all the sacrifices she and my dad had made for me, and said that she couldn't believe that this was how I chose to repay them. All of my self-respect went down the tubes. I felt engulfed by guilt. When I was in their house, I felt like my presence sickened them. I was under so much stress from the pregnancy that I couldn't take it anymore. I told them I was going to move in with Eric and his father. They begged me not to leave, and so I stayed for a while, but it was unbearable. They refused to let me be alone with Eric. We continued to fight, but the power-struggle ended on the night my dad cut my hair because I'd been caught at the mall with Eric. At that point, I realized I couldn't live with the pressure and the guilt.

The first chance I had, I packed my stuff and moved out while my parents were at a company picnic. I left a message on their answering machine stating that I was gone and not to look for me. I moved in with Eric and his dad. I still, to this day, cannot believe I did that, but his family offered me whatever I needed.

From the time I was pregnant, I just absolutely fell in love with the baby. I wanted to give it everything that I possibly could. After I started checking into things, I realized that I wouldn't be able to give him all those things. If I could've raised him on love, I would've done it in a heartbeat. But I know that it takes so much more to make a child happy. Growing up with a mom and dad is something that I don't take for granted because I have a lot of friends who don't have that same luxury, and I really think that is something that's important. That's when I thought about adoption.

Finding an Option

The real inspiration came from a family that I baby-sat for. They had a little girl, and I took care of her a lot. I just loved her to death. And they were just the perfect family; we really got close. The dad would give me a ride home, and we'd talk about all kinds of stuff. When I told him I was pregnant, he told me that his little girl was adopted through a place called the Gladney Center in Fort Worth, Texas. That young mother had been in the same position that I was in. I saw what a wonderful life her little girl had now, and so I thought it would be possible for my baby to have the same kind of life.

I called the Gladney Center and found out that they had a high school on campus, only for pregnant girls choosing adoption, which appealed to me because I didn't want to go to public school while I was pregnant. I was too ashamed. At the Center, you could take a pillow to class if you needed it. If you were sick, you could make up the work when you felt better. There were dormitories where we slept and a cafeteria for meals. They also staffed trained counselors to help prepare us for the grief we would face. As long as you place your baby up for adoption, there is no charge to stay at the center, not even for medical bills. All of this came as a great relief after the chaos I'd been experiencing. After visiting the campus, Eric and I decided that it was the right place.

That fall, about five months into my pregnancy, I ended up going to the Gladney Center and living there. It was about an hour from my house. The people there were so caring and they knew what I was going through.

The greatest comfort came from the girls there who made me realize that I wasn't alone, and I wasn't the only one to make a mistake. Some of the girls there were struggling more with the idea of giving up their babies for adoption. A lot of their worries were cleared up by the counseling, but a friend of mine there ended up leaving because she realized she couldn't go through with the adoption. But for the most part, all the girls supported each other and offered reassurance. It was a good environment.

Choosing the Right Family

While I was there, I made a list of things that I wanted my child to have in his adopted family. In that list, I put that I wanted the parents to be married for at least four years. I wanted them to have a stable relationship and to be financially stable as well. And I wanted a big extended family close by, lots of aunts and uncles and grandparents. I wanted the family to have pets. I wanted them to be able to go on vacations, and I wanted them to be Baptists.

Once the Gladney Center had my list, they presented me with three files. All of them were just incredible, but one couple matched every request I had made. I read a letter they wrote, and I looked at pictures and I got descriptions of them. He's a businessman, and she's an elementary school principal. They live on a river and have about two acres of land. They wrote that the child they'd adopt would have lots of trees to climb and lots of pets. They had everything that I wanted for him. . . .

Eric was there when I was in labor. His family was there too. I thought the labor was very hard. It lasted about 13 hours.

After the baby was born, I wanted to meet the couple I had chosen. They got him that morning, and then I met with them after that. By law, you have to wait six days before you can sign. You have to go to court. After you've relinquished all your rights [to the child], they give the baby to the parents.

It was so special meeting them. It was so neat to be able to look into their eyes and tell them how much I loved him. And to hear from them how much they loved him and what they wanted to do for him. They named him Richard Dillon. They call him Dillon.

I gave them a baby book and asked them to fill it out and send it back to me. After Dillon's first birthday, I got it back. Inside it, they wrote things that he'd said and done, and it's really special to me. They're so great. They're the best people. I also sent them an album of Eric and me. It's full of pictures of us from when we were babies and growing up, so that Dillon will know exactly what we look like. He can compare his photos to ours and see who he looks like. I also wrote him a letter telling him why I did the things that I did and why I made the choice that I did, and I hope he'll always know how much I love him.

Rebuilding My Life

I stayed at the Gladney Center after the baby was born because I wanted to finish out the semester. It worked out perfectly. I started school there, then I had the baby . . . , then we had Christmas break and I had about two weeks to go back and finish up.

I moved back home after I finished school. It was really hard being back home, away from Eric. That first Christmas was just unreal. My parents were understanding, but they still didn't want me to be alone with Eric. I really needed him more than anything then. I realize that they were just trying to protect me from more pain, but they were so strict with me. There was still a lot of tension between us. It took a long time for me to regain their trust.

Adoption May Benefit Pregnant Teenagers

Adolescent mothers who place their newborns for adoption are more likely than those who rear their infants to experience regret over their decision one year after the birth. However, according to a study of pregnant and postpartum teenagers in Ohio, these reactions are not associated with higher levels of depression or diminished feelings of efficacy. Moreover, adolescents who choose adoption complete more education, have higher rates of employment and lower rates of welfare receipt, and engage in less sexual risk-taking than do teenagers who keep their infants.

K. Mahler, *Family Planning Perspectives*, 1997.

Going back to public school was awkward. When I left, no one knew what had happened, and when I came back, pretty much everyone knew where I'd been, and if they didn't, then they found out. But no matter how hard things got for me, I always felt like I made the right choice. I knew, without a doubt in my mind, that it was the right decision to make. And everyone that said anything to me said something positive, and anyone who had something bad to say didn't say anything to my face. But I was never the same after that.

I was 10 times more mature than the other girls there. I remember sitting in class listening to them talk about boyfriend problems, and I'd think to myself, 'Well, I just had a baby and gave it up for adoption.' Their problems just seemed so minor compared to what I'd been through.

As far as boys and dating, I was still seeing Eric when I went back to school in January. We were together until March. I sometimes felt uncomfortable around other guys because I worried that they might be judging me. I did have a boyfriend my senior year who knew all about what had happened. It's sometimes hard for me to know in a relationship when it is the right time for me to tell someone about it. I have some friends who don't know about this.

Looking Ahead

I hope there will be a time when Dillon and I can get to know each other. There is a registry. When he's 21, I can sign the registry. If he signs it also, if it's a mutual thing, then it can be arranged for us to meet. I think that his adoptive parents will be fine with that.

Dillon already knows that he's adopted. He's three now. From the time they first held him in their arms, they told him that he was adopted, so there will never be any point in his life that he's surprised about it. That's something that is done in almost all adoptive situations these days. It's not the kind of thing that you just sit someone down and tell them when they're a certain age. That could be really traumatic.

The whole situation for me is bittersweet. I know that I wouldn't be where I am today if all these things hadn't happened in my life. I would've gotten in a lot more trouble probably. It turned my life around. I went through a lot of things with my parents. I went through a lot of pain. Things are mended with my family now. Eric and I still keep in touch even though my parents still don't like him. He called the other day. Every time I get pictures I try to get in contact with him. Our lives are really different now. He's married, and I'm in college. I have lots of friends and I'm doing well.

Still, I wouldn't wish the situation I was in on anyone at any time. I think it's so important that teenagers understand what they're getting into when they have sex, especially when they are that young. I had no clue. I feel that I got in this situation because I was too afraid to talk to somebody. I didn't feel I could talk to my parents. There were plenty of other people around that I could've talked to, but I was too afraid. I just couldn't do it. Now I know that if I had confided in somebody, everything could've been a lot different."

| *"Promoting adoption instead of abortion sounds life-affirming, but it's actually physically dangerous, cruel and punitive."*

Adoption May Not Be an Option for Pregnant Teenagers

Katha Pollitt

Many politicians and public figures tout adoption as the humanitarian alternative to abortion. In the following viewpoint, Katha Pollitt argues that such ideology is damaging to pregnant teenagers who may suffer serious physical and emotional repercussions from carrying a pregnancy to term at such a young age. She maintains that instilling guilt in young girls who choose abortion instead of adoption revives the negative social stigma of teenage pregnancy that prevailed in the 1950s and 1960s. Pollitt is a columnist with *Nation*, a weekly journal of political and social issues.

As you read, consider the following questions:
1. How does Pollitt define the welfare family cap?
2. What differences between the United States' and Europe's policies on teenage sexuality does the author describe?
3. According to the author, how were girls coerced to choose adoption in the 1950s and 1960s?

As the "family values"/teen-sex/abortion debate winds on with no end in sight, adoption is being touted as a rare area of consensus: the way to discourage "illegitimacy" while providing poor children with stable homes, the peace pipe in the abortion wars. Whatever may be the difficulties and conflicts of actual people involved in the adoption triangle, at the political level, it's all win-win: adoption and apple pie.

Whenever I question the facile promotion of adoption as a solution to the problem du jour I get angry letters from adoptive parents. So I want to be clear: Of course adoption can be a wonderful thing; of course the ties between adoptive parents and children are as profound as those between biological ones. But can't one both rejoice in the happiness adoption can bring to individuals and ask hard questions about the social functions it is being asked to fill? I can't be the only person who has noticed that the Clinton Administration which supports the family cap—the denial of a modest benefit increase to women who conceive an additional child while on welfare—would bestow on all but the richest families a $5,000 tax credit to defray the costs of adoption. Thus, the New Jersey baby who is deemed unworthy of $64 a month, or $768 a year, in government support if he stays in his family of origin immediately becomes six times more valuable once he joins a supposedly better-ordered household. Maybe unwed mothers should trade kids.

In 1995, mass adoption was supposed to rescue innocent babies from the effects of defunding their guilty teenage mothers—a bizarre brainstorm . . . that has fortunately faded for now. In 1996, adoption is back in a more accustomed role, as an "alternative" to abortion—a notion long supported by abortion-rights opponents . . . , and recently picked up by some pro-choicers too. The wrong women insisting on their right to have children, the right women refusing to—it's hard to avoid the conclusion that as public policy, adoption is being pushed as a way of avoiding hard questions about class and sex. After all, if poverty is the problem, we could enable mothers and children to live decently, as is done throughout Western Europe. If teenage pregnancy is the problem, we could insist on contraception, sex education and health care—the approach that has also worked very well in Western Europe, where teens are about as sexually active as they are in this country, but where rates of teen pregnancy range from half of ours (England and Wales) to one-tenth (the Netherlands).

Problems with Adoption

Advocates for adoption as a solution to childbearing among unwed teens ignore a number of inconvenient facts. For example, most infertile couples seeking to adopt are white, and most of them wish to adopt only healthy white newborns. (An estimated half-million children are living in foster care, but there is little political pressure to make these children available for adoption, because they are the wrong color, the wrong age, and the wrong class.) But white teenage mothers—who in 1992 accounted for about 60 percent of teens giving birth out of wedlock—are more likely than black teenage mothers to marry after the birth of a child and to be living with the father of their baby at the time of the birth, making them unlikely candidates to relinquish their children. Thus, if more women gave up their children for adoption, there would simply be more children in foster care, since many of them would be black and the adoption market for such children is limited.

Kristin Luker, *Dubious Conceptions: The Politics of Teenage Pregnancy*, 1996.

How much sense does adoption make as a large-scale alternative to abortion? Journalists constantly cite the National Council for Adoption's (NCA) claim that 1–2 million Americans wish to adopt—which would make between twenty and forty potential adopters for every one of the 50,000 or so non-kin adoptions formalized in a typical year. But what is this estimate based on? According to the NCA, it's a rough extrapolation from figures on infertility, and includes anyone who makes any gesture in the direction of adoption—even a phone call which means they are counting most of my women friends, some of the men. . . . The number of serious, viable candidates is bound to be much smaller: For all the publicity surrounding their tragic circumstances, in 1995 Americans adopted only 2,193 Chinese baby girls. Even if there were no other objections, the adoption and abortion numbers are too incommensurate for the former to be a real "alternative" to the latter.

But of course, there are other objections. There are good reasons why only 3 percent of white girls and 1 percent of black girls—and an even tinier percentage of adult women—choose adoption. Maybe more would do so if adoption were more fluid and open—a kind of open-ended "guardianship" arrangement, but that would surely discourage potential adoptive parents. The glory days of white-baby relinquishment in the 1950s and 1960s depended on coercion—the illegality of abortion, the sexual double standard and the stigma of unwed motherhood, enforced by family, neighbors, school, social work, medicine, church, law. Those girls gave up their babies because they had no choice and that's why we are now hearing from so many sad and furious 50-year-old birth mothers. Do we really want to create a new generation of them by applying the guilt and pressure tactics that a behavior change of such magnitude would require?

Right now, pregnant girls and women are free to make an adoption plan, and for some it may indeed be the right choice. But why persuade more to—unless one espouses the anti-choice philosophy that even the fertilized egg has a right to be born, and that terminating a pregnancy is "selfish"? I'm not belittling the longings of would-be adoptive parents, but theirs is not a problem a teenager should be asked to solve. Pregnancy and childbirth are immense events, physically, emotionally, socially, with lifelong effects; it isn't selfish to say no to them.

Promoting adoption instead of abortion sounds life-affirming, but it's actually physically dangerous, cruel and punitive. That's why the political and media figures now supporting it wouldn't dream of urging it on their own daughters. . . . They have a right to put themselves first.

Periodical Bibliography

The following articles have been selected to supplement the diverse views presented in this chapter.

Spencer Abraham and Mary Landrieu	"Promoting Adoption: A No-Lose Proposition," *Christian Science Monitor*, May 15, 1998.
Alan Guttmacher Institute	"Teenagers' Pregnancy Intentions and Decisions: A Study of Young Women in California Choosing to Give Birth," 1999.
Amy Bach	"No Choice for Teens," *Nation*, October 11, 1999.
Christine Granados	"Young, Single . . . and a Mom: Latina Mothers Build Personal Strength from Life," *Hispanic*, June 1997.
Yvette R. Harris	"Adolescent Abortion," *Society*, July/August 1997.
Nancy K.S. Hochman	"For Whom the Bells Toll," *Seventeen*, October 1998.
Marguerite Kelly	"The Angles on Single Motherhood," *Washington Post*, May 14, 2001.
K. Mahler	"Young Mothers Who Choose Adoption May Be Regretful, but Not Usually Depressed," *Family Planning Perspectives*, May/June 1997.
Marshall H. Medoff	"An Estimate of Teenage Abortion Demand," *Journal of Socio-Economics*, March/April 1999.
Lauren Mills	"Promises to Keep," *Good Housekeeping*, May 2000.
M.L. O'Connor	"Women Who Were Born to Teenage Mothers Have Nearly Double the Risk of Childbearing," *Family Planning Perspectives*, September/October, 1997.
James Ragland	"Teen Mom Accepts Challenge," *Dallas Morning News*, June 22, 2001.
Katharine Q. Seelye	"Concealing a Pregnancy to Avoid Telling Mom," *New York Times*, June 15, 1997.
Annette Tomal	"The Effect of Religious Membership on Teenage Abortion Rates," *Journal of Youth and Adolescence*, February 2001.

CHAPTER 4

How Can Teenage Pregnancy Be Reduced?

Chapter Preface

The 1996 Welfare Reform Act contains many provisions aimed at combating teenage pregnancy, including the reduction of welfare benefits for teens who are not in school and not living with a suitable guardian and increased enforcement of statutory rape laws. One of the most controversial provisions provides $50 million in federal funds for abstinence-only sex education in schools.

Supporters of abstinence-only sex education maintain that traditional sex education programs, which provide information about contraception and protection from disease, send students mixed messages about whether sexual activity is permissible at such a young age. The 1996 act requires that abstinence-only sex education programs convey to students that "abstinence from sexual activity outside marriage is the expected standard for all school-age children," and "sexual activity outside of the context of marriage is likely to have harmful psychological and physical effects." As stated by medical doctor Joe McIlhaney, "The best that 'safer sex' approaches can offer is some risk reduction. Abstinence . . . offers risk elimination. When the risks of pregnancy and disease are so great, even with contraception, how can we advocate anything less?"

Others maintain that abstinence-only sex education programs are unrealistic. Since many adolescents are having sex, these critics argue, teens should be informed of how to protect themselves against pregnancy and sexually transmitted infections. Traditional sex education programs advocate abstinence as the ideal way to avoid pregnancy and infection, but also teach students various methods of birth control and how to use them correctly. According to Debra W. Haffner, president of the Sexuality Information and Education Council of the United States, "There is no question that young people want help saying no. . . . But we must do much more. Teens also need information about their bodies, gender roles, sexual abuse, pregnancy and STD prevention."

The effectiveness of abstinence-only education is one of the issues discussed in the following chapter on measures to reduce teen pregnancy.

> *"Abstinence can and should be taught not only as the cornerstone of sex education but as a lifestyle to be mastered."*

Abstinence-Only Sex Education Can Reduce Teenage Pregnancy

Lakita Garth

In an effort to reduce the high rates of teenage pregnancy in the United States, political, religious, and educational leaders have implemented sex education programs that focus on abstinence. Traditional sex education programs describe various methods of birth control and ways to prevent sexually transmitted infections. Abstinence-only education programs state that abstinence until marriage is the standard for human sexual behavior and warn students of the psychological and physical harms that may accompany premarital sex. In the following viewpoint, Lakita Garth makes this argument and contends that abstinence teaches students the fundamental life lessons of "self-control, self-discipline, and delay of self-gratification." Garth is a noted speaker on various issues such as race relations, politics, feminism, AIDS, abortion, and is one of the country's leading abstinence advocates.

As you read, consider the following questions:
1. According to the author, what did the young mothers at the Simpson Alternative School want to know more about?
2. How does Garth differentiate between sexually experienced and sexually active?
3. What does the author claim is the greatest determinant of women leaving the welfare system?

Excerpted from Lakita Garth's testimony before the Empowerment Subcommittee of the Small Business Committee, July 16, 1998.

I am a '20-something' year old black female, a former 2nd-runner up to Miss Black America, an entertainer, president of a corporation, and a virgin. I've had the unique opportunity to be invited by School Districts, Abstinence groups, and even state organizations such as the Department of Health and Human Services and Office of Family Planning in California, to share the message of abstinence. I've spoken to nearly a million teenagers of different racial and socio-economic backgrounds in assemblies across America over the past 9 years. My greatest motivation in doing so is to empower them with some of the same tools I was fortunate enough to grow up with, which I feel are lacking in our culture today. The first thing I communicate to teens and adults alike is the fact that abstinence is not just shaking ones finger at a generation and telling them to 'just say no' to sex. Abstinence is a lifestyle. It is mastering the art of:

1. Self-control
2. Self-discipline
3. Delay of self-gratification . . .

To more vividly share what I have witnessed over these past few years, I'd like to put it in the context of the 10 most commonly shared opinions about teens and sexuality:

1. It can't happen to me
2. We just need to teach them safe sex
3. They're gonna do it anyway
4. Sex is a natural bodily function that can't be controlled
5. It's too late to teach them abstinence
6. Well, I think as long as you love the person, it's perfectly okay
7. Kids will never buy into an abstinence message
8. Hey, if it feels good, do it
9. You should be able to do whatever you want as long as you don't hurt anybody
10. What people do behind closed doors is nobody else's business

It Can Happen to Anyone

It can't happen to me—is perhaps the prevailing attitude of most every teenager in America regardless of what era they grew up in. It is from this attitude that I have found that all the other presuppositions stem. However, it is important to take a brief look at how prevalent the negative consequences of promiscuity among teens has increased over the past few decades.

- The teen birthrate in the United States is the highest of any industrialized nation, nearly twice as great as that of the United Kingdom and 15 times that of Japan.
- 1 million teenage girls get pregnant each year. Of that, approximately 40% will receive government assistance.
- 33,000 people contract an STD everyday. Approximately 2/3 are under the age of 25.
- 50% of the sexually active single adult population has, or will have, at least 1 STD in their lifetime.
- AIDS is the leading killer of Americans between the ages of 25 and 44.
- Nearly 40 million surgical abortions have been performed in America since the *Roe vs. Wade* decision in 1973.
- Illegitimate births have increased 400% since 1963, the historical date that marks the beginning of the sexual revolution. . . .

We just need to teach them how to be safe—I rarely hear this from teens anymore and I'm hearing it less and less from adults. Is the lack of information and the unavailability of contraception the reason for the present state of illegitimacy and rising STD rates among teens? Not in my experience. Among my visits to homes for unwed mothers and 'pregnant schools' such as Simpson Alternative School in Chicago, I found some very consistent traits. None of the girls said their pregnancies were due to ignorance of contraception methods. As a matter of fact, only 14% of teens don't use birth control because they lack knowledge of or access to birth control.

Moreover, many admitted that they had intentionally gotten pregnant, and when I asked how many of them were using "protection" (condoms, the pill, etc.) when they conceived, on average 3–4 out of 10 raised their hands. By the way, what were those contraception failure rates again?

Upon witnessing this, I thought it would be interesting to ask them a similar question Eunice Kennedy Shriver asked when she visited a group of teen mothers.

"What do you want to know more about?" Surprisingly every group of teen mothers I spoke with responded the same way they responded to her. The majority asked questions such as, "How do I live an abstinent lifestyle?" Furthermore, I have no recollection of any pregnant girls ever asking me about better contraception devices. . . .

Teen Sex Is Unacceptable

They're gonna do it anyway—Is what an assistant vice principal told me before I spoke in her school. In fact this is perhaps the most quoted response I hear adults say when commenting on teen sexuality. I often wonder why that is. We don't seem to have that same attitude towards teens when it comes to other risky behaviors. We communicate that drugs, alcohol, and violence are not acceptable and even make the effort to inform them that these behaviors are not only socially unacceptable but illegal as well. Why haven't we done this in regard to sex?

We haven't clearly communicated that teen sexual involvement is an unacceptable behavior because we've sent a mixed message. Granted everyone isn't going to abstain, and provision must be made for those who have deviated from the standard. However, we have made the exception the rule and now the standard, sexual abstinence, has become the exception. We must be just as consistent in the messages we communicate to teens in regards to sex as we've been with drugs and violence. . . .

Sex is a natural bodily function that can't be controlled— Is what a fellow guest on a talk show told me and amazingly enough has been the prevailing attitude when it comes to teaching anything about sex. It can best be summarized by a quote from Dr. Ruth. 'Asking young people to control their libido is asking them too much. Their libido is too strong.' If sex is an uncontrollable bodily function such as breathing, sleeping, eating, or even going to the restroom then it would be safe to assume somehow that if one were prevented from exercising these functions, detrimental side effects would occur, or even death. However, after engaging in some research, I've not yet found a documented case or an obituary that read, "Johnny . . . 17 years old . . . cause of death . . . virginity."

I always get a response of laughter when I share this widely held opinion of teens. DuSable High School in Chicago was no exception. Principle Mingo told me that his high school was the first Chicago City School to have a school based clinic implemented, it was known as the worst school in America in the early 90's, and is currently one of the 3 poorest high schools in the country. After receiving a standing ovation from the student body after a 75 minute abstinence presentation a young boy from DuSable High School responded to this attitude best with the affirmation of his peers standing by. He said, "If they can potty train us growing up and expect to use self-control when we're older why can't they have the same expectation when it comes to sex. What do they think we are, animals?". . .

Best Friends

Is teaching abstinence realistic? You bet. Let me highlight just one approach: the young women involved in the Best Friends program, founded in Washington 10 years ago. Beginning in the fifth grade and continuing through high school, girls are provided adult mentors, fun activities and social support for abstaining from sex, drugs and alcohol and finishing their education. The focus is on freedom for the future gained by delaying what might feel good now but damages lives later. A 1995 study found that girls in the Best Friends program had a 1.1 percent pregnancy rate, compared with a 26 percent rate for teen girls in the Washington area.

Joe McIlhaney, *Insight on the News*, September 29, 1997.

It's too late to teach them abstinence—is what I heard a Baltimore, Maryland high school principle say on ABC's Primetime with Diane Sawyer. She like many others has come to equate sexual experience with being sexually active. I've often debated officials, who've said, "Look, over 50% of high school students are sexually active by the time they graduate, why are you wasting your time?" This commonly used percentage is misleading. Although over half of teens may have had sex, that does not mean that they currently are sexually active. Many of these young people express how they have had sex a few or several times and then stopped because the experience was not as they say, "all that."

Let's take a deeper look at this line of reasoning. In the 60's many young people engaged in drug experimentation —you may even know of a few. But did anyone say that it was too late to discourage this addictive and dangerous behavior? No, as a matter of fact most of them not only stopped but became productive members of society—and even politicians. Is it either fair or accurate to say that these individuals are still active drug users because they have used drugs in the past? No. Then it is never too late to encourage teens to stop engaging in risky behaviors. . . .

Heart Issues

Well, I think as long as you love the person, it's perfectly okay. That's what Damien Harris told me the father of her son, Gregory, said to her before she got pregnant. Damien was also [a part of] the statistic that children of adolescent mothers also become adolescent mothers. Three days after Damien was born her mother walked out of the hospital and was never seen again. Although her parents were never married, she was raised with her paternal grandmother in Los Angeles, California. She was a gifted artist on her way to college until she got pregnant and ended up on government assistance. Soon after her son was born she moved in with me, and an abstinent lifestyle was one of the many things I began to encourage her to practice. We lived together for several years during which she got off government assistance, got a full ride scholarship to Long Beach State University, moved into her own apartment and got married. While living together she shared many things with me in hopes that no other girl would follow the path she took as a teenager. She has said many times that she knew about and used contraception but still she contracted STDs and got pregnant. She believes that many are quick to push safe sex on inner-city girls but never truly address the heart issues of why they are having sex.

Now she is an advocate of abstinence until marriage and regrets not having waited until she got married. Even though the greatest determinant of women leaving the welfare system is marriage, not training programs, still marriage is rarely encouraged in sex ed classes (especially in the inner cities). Fortunately, Damien . . . has surpassed the low expectations placed upon black females and broken the statistics. I got to participate in her wedding last year, and as I saw her son Gregory walk down the isle as the ring bearer I had never remembered seeing him happier. He told me, "Aunt Kita, mommy and I are getting married today!" Now Gregory has something most little boys in the African-American community will never have, a father who lives at home.

Kids will never buy into an abstinence message—was what I was initially told by a public relations firm in Los Angeles that was contracted by the state of California to promote The Partnership for Responsible Parenting. But they soon began to change their minds when I toured the state with the Office of Family Planning speaking to hundreds of high school students. Eric Curren, Senior Account Executive, for the public relations firm, said he "had a blast and being back in the office hasn't been the same." He's received responses from all over the state and the responses were over whelming. "The claim that students are unwilling to listen to an abstinence message is untrue . . . they eagerly participated. . They thought it was cool." He said teen "surveys showed that students were not only receptive to the abstinence message, but that they were thankful for it: 'I'm glad somebody said what I already thought: You don't have to do it to be cool.'" Eric and others on the tour said the message of self-control, self-discipline, and the delay of self-gratification was "empowering.". . .

Casualties of the Sexual Revolution

Hey, if it feels good, do it—was the mantra of the 60's. Just as it is known that marijuana in the 60's is not like marijuana in the 90's, so sex in the 60's is not like sex in the 90's. What was sown to the wind is now reaping the whirlwind. In the 60's sex was questioned by a generation of boomers as an issue of morality. The culture formerly had standards and this generation, knowing what the standards were, challenged them by engaging in what the dictionary calls immorality—defying a known moral law. These same individuals grew up and became parents to children who are now amoral—without knowledge of any moral code—in regards to their sexual behavior. Thus, I am a product of an amoral generation known as X and my counterpart known as the Milliniels. In 1966, the then Executive Director of SIECUS (Sexuality Information and Education Council of the United States) asked, "What is sex for? It's for fun. . . We need new values to establish when and how we should have sexual experiences."

Well, we got what we asked for, and that's why you're reading this paper. Some, however, are still fighting for a free sex crusade that has proven not to be free at all because everybody is paying—financially, socially, emotionally, physically, and some even with their own lives. Every revolution has its casualties, and although there have been personal victories, can we honestly say that we have won the war? Before answering yes, please remember that it is mine and the subsequent generation that have suffered the greatest amount of casualties. For my peers and I, sex isn't merely a moral question but a question of "Is it worth the hassle?" And today, unlike that carefree frolic in the grass in Woodstock days, it's a matter of life and death. As one high school boy put it, "Sex doesn't feel good when you're dead.". . .

Times have changed and I think we've seen the effects of a culture that has aggressively hailed the anthem of "if it feels good do it." Change, however, is in the wind and if we listen closely to the chorus of voices growing louder among the youth, and not dimmer with age, it is obvious that a generation "after Woodstock, a new youth rebellion is afoot. The anthem of this new generation: True Love Waits," [according to] Cheryl Wetstein, [author of an article published in the *Washington Times* titled] "With Groups' Help, Teens Take Pride in Virginity."

The Social Costs of Teen Pregnancy

You should be able to do whatever you want as long as you don't hurt anybody—a Chief District Court Judge for the 5th Judicial District of North Carolina who served on the National Council for juvenile and family court judges doesn't think so. Judge Gilbert H. Burnett told me during a lunch meeting that during his 23 years judging criminals and juveniles he believes that the biggest cause of crime, public health costs, and welfare is adolescent pregnancy. He believes that if teen pregnancies could be cut in half that we would see a decline in crime, public health costs, and welfare within 12 years. Every year:

- One million teenage girls get pregnant each year. Out of that million: one-third have induced abortions, 14% miscarry, and 52% give birth. Out of that 52%, 80% is in poverty and end up on public assistance.
- The daughters of adolescent mothers are more likely to become adolescent moms themselves, and the sons are more likely to wind up in prison.
- If a teenage girl gives birth to a male child, the chances are three times as great that he will end up in prison when he is older. Whereas, if the circumstances were identical, but she waited until she was 22 or 23 there is ⅓ less chance he would end up in prison.
- An estimated $1 billion is spent annually in the construction and maintenance of criminal facilities. In which close to 70% that are incarcerated come from single parent homes. . . .

What people do behind closed doors is nobody else's business—If this is true then why do these same people come from behind closed doors and expect the rest of society to pay for their "behind closed door activity?" Certainly, we all concede that you can't legislate morality, however, you can legislate moral laws. For every law inherently sets a standard and an expectation of behavior. Recently, Judge Burnett had a conversation with a local pediatrician who told him that 80% of the babies born in his hospital, who are on life support, were born to teenage mothers. Some of the costs can run as much as $600,000 per infant, which of course is passed on to others who are to stay out of their "business." "We must discourage sexual activity among youth. . . The younger teens start having sex, the more partners they will have which automatically . . . [puts them] more at risk for contracting STDs. . . .

Teaching Necessary Life Skills

After engaging hundreds of thousands of teens across America, I've yet to receive a negative response from a student (the person whom this message directly affects). Abstinence can and should be taught not only as the cornerstone of sex education but as a lifestyle to be mastered. What plausible argument could anyone give for rejecting the priority of teaching self-control, self-discipline, and the delay of self-gratification? Is it possible that we have neglected these necessary life skills? When I ask teens if perhaps this is true, the overwhelming majority seems to think so. . . .

Discouraging sexual activity among teens, not accommodating it as we have [been] should be the priority. Permissiveness and an undisciplined lifestyle has never and never will produce sustained excellence or success. Much to my surprise I even found an unlikely advocate of teen abstinence, none other than talk show host, Jerry Springer, who earlier this summer was thunderously applauded by his audience. He has stated several times, "Teenagers have no business having sex at all!" Even Jerry Springer stumbled upon this revelation. When will we?

> *"Abstinence-only sexuality education fails to provide adolescents with the information they need to protect their health and well-being."*

Abstinence-Only Sex Education Cannot Reduce Teenage Pregnancy

National Abortion and Reproductive Rights Action League

Many people argue that traditional sex education, which promotes abstinence but also teaches students about contraception and protection against sexually transmitted infections, is confusing to students. These people contend that this method of instruction encourages students to have sex and risk teenage pregnancy. In the following viewpoint, the National Abortion and Reproductive Rights Action League (NARAL) argues that teaching students about birth control and protection provides students with essential information about their health and sexuality. NARAL is a political organization dedicated to preserving the right to choose while promoting policies and programs that help to make abortion less necessary.

As you read, consider the following questions:

1. According to the author, how do the rates of teenage sex in the Netherlands, Germany, and France compare with the United States?
2. What are the functions of the Adolescent Family Life Act, as described by NARAL?
3. What does the author claim are some of the shortcomings of abstinence-only education?

R ecently abstinence-only education has captivated the attention of legislators. Through welfare reform legislation that establishes an abstinence-only education entitlement program and appropriations for the Adolescent Family Life Act program (AFLA), Congress has allocated millions of dollars for abstinence-only education.

Such an emphasis on abstinence-only education is misplaced. Abstinence-only programs stress that abstinence is the only acceptable behavior for adolescents. They fail to provide information regarding pregnancy, sexually transmitted disease (STD) and human immunodeficiency virus (HIV) prevention beyond urging that teenagers abstain. Often, such programs stress abstinence until marriage. They frequently base their message on fear, using scare tactics rather than factual, medically accurate information to educate. If information regarding contraception or STD/HIV prevention methods other than abstinence is included, such information generally includes only failure rates.

Comprehensive, responsible sexuality education, on the other hand, not only teaches abstinence and resistance skills, but also provides teens with the contraceptive and STD/HIV prevention information they need to make responsible decisions if and when they become sexually active. Although abstinence is a vital component of a comprehensive sexuality education program, it should not be the only lesson taught. By denying teens the full range of information regarding human sexuality, abstinence-only sexuality education fails to provide adolescents with the information they need to protect their health and well-being.

An Adolescent Reproductive Health Crisis

Despite the positive trends identified in recent surveys, the U.S. continues to face a crisis in adolescent reproductive health. Although some statistics demonstrate a decline in teen sexual activity, a decline in teen pregnancy, and an increase in contraceptive use at first sexual intercourse, other statistics present a bleaker view. Consider these facts:

- More than half of all teens aged 15 to 19 years old in the U.S. have had sexual intercourse.
- The percentage of teen girls who have engaged in sex-

ual intercourse before age 15 has risen from 11 percent in 1988 to 19 percent in 1995.

- While the percentage of teens who used contraception at first intercourse has increased in recent years, the percentage of teens who used contraception at last intercourse has *decreased.* Findings from one survey demonstrate that fewer than half of all never-married teen males aged 15 to 19 who have had sex used condoms every time they had sex during the last year. Moreover, the likelihood that a teen male will use a condom 100 percent of the time tends to decrease with age.
- Nationally each year, almost one million teenagers get pregnant, and more than three-fourths of all teen pregnancies are unintended.
- Annually in the U.S., three million teens are newly infected with a sexually transmitted disease, and one in every three sexually active individuals will contract a STD by age 24.
- One in four new cases of HIV infection befalls someone younger than 22 years of age.
- Adolescents often receive inadequate prenatal care and give birth to over 46,000 low birthweight babies each year.
- Compared to adolescents who commonly receive open and frank media messages and education concerning sexuality and safe sex in the Netherlands, Germany, and France, American teens initiate sexual intercourse at a younger age and use oral contraceptives less. In addition, American teens experience higher rates of birth, abortion, and some sexually transmitted diseases than their European counterparts. . . .

The Rise of Abstinence-Only Education

The emphasis on only abstinence in sexuality education has taken a variety of forms.

- In 1996, Congress passed welfare reform legislation that established an abstinence-only education entitlement program. Administered through the Maternal and Child Health Block Grant (MCHBG) program, this legislation allocates federal funds to programs that have abstinence education as their "exclusive purpose." Beginning in fiscal year 1998, this program provides $50 million in grant money each year for five years. Participating states must match every four dollars of federal grant money with three dollars of non-federal funds. All 50 states applied for the fiscal year (FY) 1998 funds, although officials in New Hampshire and California ultimately declined the funding for FY 1998.

Under the federal law, the term "abstinence education" means an educational or motivational program which:

- "has as its exclusive purpose, teaching the social, psychological, and health gains to be realized by abstaining from sexual activity;"
- "teaches abstinence from sexual activity outside marriage as the expected standard for all school age children;"
- "teaches that abstinence from sexual activity is the only certain way to avoid out-of-wedlock pregnancy, sexually transmitted diseases, and other associated health problems;"
- "teaches that a mutually faithful monogamous relationship in context of marriage is the expected standard of human sexual activity;"
- "teaches that sexual activity outside of the context of marriage is likely to have harmful psychological and physical effects;"
- "teaches that bearing children out-of-wedlock is likely to have harmful consequences for the child, the child's parents, and society;"
- "teaches young people how to reject sexual advances and how alcohol and drug use increases vulnerability to sexual advances;" and
- "teaches the importance of attaining self-sufficiency before engaging in sexual activity."

- The Adolescent Family Life Act (AFLA) also provides federal funds to support education programs that teach abstinence. Enacted in 1981, the AFLA program provides grants to public and nonprofit organizations to support abstinence education and programs that provide direct services for pregnant and parenting teens. For FY 1998 Congress appropriated $16.709 million for AFLA, compared to $6.250 million for FY 1994, an increase of 167 percent.

- The emphasis that Congress has placed on abstinence-only education sets a bad precedent for the states, possibly draining money and energy from comprehensive sexuality education programs. Only 20 states, including the District of Columbia, require schools to provide sexuality education. Of those 20 states, only ten require that sexuality education teach abstinence and provide information about contraception. In 1998 alone, states enacted 14 new laws (three of which are resolutions) which focus on abstinence-only or abstinence-until-marriage education.

Failing to Provide Necessary Information

Abstinence education is an essential part of sexuality education. Adolescents should be encouraged to avoid premature sexual involvement, and sexuality education should teach respect for others and prepare teens to deal with peer pressure and pressure from partners to engage in sexual activity. Yet abstinence should not be the only lesson taught. Teens need to learn how to protect themselves if they become sexually active.

Although as a general matter parents should have the primary responsibility of teaching their children about the risks and responsibilities of sexual activity and how to prevent unintended pregnancy and sexually transmitted diseases, many parents do not provide sexuality education at home. A recent survey by the Kaiser Family Foundation and ABC Television found that only 52 percent of parents with at least one child aged eight to 18 said they have ever talked to him or her about the "importance of using protection, such as condoms, to prevent pregnancy or disease if they become sexually active." Many parents lack the information to teach these lessons and cannot explain STDs and contraception to their children. Others may feel uncomfortable discussing sex or may deny that their children are sexually active. A mere 11 percent of teens receive most of their STD information from parents and others in the family. In addition, some teens simply are not receptive to communicating with their parents about sex.

While schools and families fail to provide adolescents with important information on sexuality, the media presents them with distorted messages about sex. A recent study found that 56 percent of television programs within a composite week contain some sexual content. Of the 1930 scenes containing sexual content, only four percent (78 scenes) incorporate any message regarding the risks or responsibilities of sexual activity, with only about half of these (41 scenes) placing a strong emphasis on such topics. In light of the facts that teens watch an average of 21 to 22 hours of television every week and that television can have a strong influence on adolescents' sexual attitudes and knowledge, these findings are particularly alarming.

The Dangers of Misinformation

As a result of shortcomings in sexuality education, family communication, and the media, teenagers often are grossly misinformed and inadequately prepared to deal with issues involving sex and may remain so throughout adulthood. For example, 40 percent of women erroneously believe that taking oral contraceptives entails greater health risks than childbearing. In addition, although at least one in four people will contract a sexually transmitted disease in their lifetime, only 14 percent of men and eight percent of women believe they are at risk. Meanwhile, when asked to list STDs they have heard of, only 13 percent of women and eight percent of men can name humanpapilloma virus (HPV), which may be the most common STD.

The lessons learned in adolescence stay with people their entire lives. By reaching adolescents, we can help reduce the number of unintended pregnancies and the need for abortion. Currently, almost 50 percent of all pregnancies in the U.S. are unintended, and over half of unintended pregnancies end in abortion.

By failing to require comprehensive, complete information about pregnancy prevention, contraception and sexually transmitted disease prevention, abstinence-only education fails to provide adolescents with the information they need to protect themselves from unintended pregnancy and disease.

Abstinence-Only Programs Are Ineffective

Not only do abstinence-only education programs fail to provide teens with the complete information they need, but evidence is lacking that they are effective in reducing teen sexual activity as well.

The National Campaign to Prevent Teen Pregnancy recently released a study which concludes that "there does not currently exist any scientifically credible, published research" that demonstrates that abstinence-only programs delay or reduce sexual activity. After reviewing six abstinence-only studies that had been published to date, the Campaign's survey finds that "[n]one of these studies found consistent and significant program effects on delaying the onset of intercourse, and at least one study provided strong evidence that the program did not delay the onset of intercourse. Thus, the weight of the evidence indicates that these abstinence programs do not delay the onset of intercourse." The report cautions, however, that "this evidence is not conclusive" due to the "significant methodological limitations" of the evaluations. The Campaign has called for "investments in high-quality program evaluation." Another review of 23 individual studies also has concluded that there is insufficient evidence to determine whether school-based abstinence-only programs delay the initiation of intercourse or affect other sexual or con-

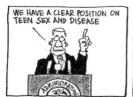
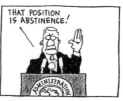
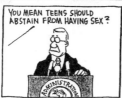
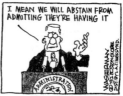

Wasserman. © 1992 by *Boston Globe*. Reprinted by permission of Los Angeles Times Syndicate.

traceptive behavior. Recently, a panel on HIV convened by the National Institute of Health criticized the MCH abstinence-only education program, stating "[a]bstinence-only programs cannot be justified in the face of effective programs and given the fact that we face an international emergency in the AIDS epidemic."

Medical Inaccuracies

Promotion of fear-based, abstinence-only curricula as the answer to the teen pregnancy problem is dangerous and counterproductive. These curricula often present misleading or medically inaccurate material, deny critical and potentially life-saving information to sexually active teens, and may even lead some to believe that precautions are futile. A Louisiana court found that portions of one such curriculum, *Sex Respect*, violated a state statute mandating that all sexuality instruction be factually accurate and religiously neutral. However, some schools still use this curriculum, which has been modified only slightly as a result of the court ruling.

More than 2500 school systems nationwide have adopted the *Sex Respect* curriculum. The curriculum contains many stereotypes and generalizations. For example, it teaches that:

> A male can experience complete sexual release with a female even if he doesn't particularly like her. A female, however, experiences more sexual fulfillment with a person she trusts and who is committed to her. . . . In most cases, girls are more interested in emotional warmth and closeness. These natural tendencies in females can, however, be weakened by a poor father-daughter relationship. Because girls who aren't on good terms with their fathers feel an unmet need for male affection, they are more likely to get involved in premarital sex.

In addition, *Sex Respect* teaches that "[i]f premarital sex came in a bottle, it would probably have to carry a Surgeon General's warning, something like the one on a package of cigarettes. There's no way to have premarital sex without hurting someone." The curriculum *Choosing the Best* actually may discourage condom use by suggesting that proper condom use is incompatible with romance. The curriculum states that "[f]or condoms to be used properly, over 10 specific steps must be followed every time which tends to minimize the romance and spontaneity of the sex act." In addition, *Choosing the Best* erroneously suggests that condoms are ineffective in preventing STDs. *Teen Aid,* another prevalent curriculum that relies heavily on scare tactics, teaches that "[s]everal factors have been advanced to explain why subsequent children [of a woman who has an abortion] are battered. Some of the mechanisms are . . . after one has aborted a child, an individual loses instinctual control over rage."

The Need for Comprehensive Sexuality Education

In addition to parents, schools also have a responsibility to provide accurate and comprehensive sexuality education. Comprehensive sexuality education should encourage young people to abstain from premature sexual involvement by acknowledging the value of abstinence while not devaluing or ignoring those young people who have had or are having sexual intercourse. Comprehensive health and sexuality education should be age and developmentally appropriate, starting early and continuing throughout school. Such education should define sexuality as a normal and healthy part of life while providing an opportunity for young people to explore their values and beliefs. It should emphasize decision-making skills and prepare teens to deal with controversial issues by supplying factually accurate information and support. It should help participants develop the self-esteem, personal responsibility, relationship skills and respect for self and others that are necessary to withstand pressure to have sex or to insist on using contraceptives and disease prevention measures if they choose to be sexually active. Such education should provide scientifically accurate information on abstinence, STD/HIV prevention methods, and contraceptive methods—including their use and effectiveness. Finally, comprehensive sexuality education should furnish information on life options for teens, including education and job planning.

Unlike the evaluations of abstinence-only programs, evaluations of comprehensive sexuality education and other programs discussing both abstinence and contraception have demonstrated positive effects. Several studies demonstrated positive outcomes such as increased knowledge, delay in onset of sex, reduction in the frequency of sex, or increased contraceptive use. For instance, the National Campaign to

Prevent Teen Pregnancy's study concludes that "[n]early all sex and AIDS education programs that have been evaluated have produced some outcome deemed socially desirable by our society." The Campaign's study also found that in-school multi-component programs, which include education and contraceptive provision, and some "community-wide" programs that focus on improved access to contraceptives and pregnancy prevention or disease prevention may increase contraceptive use and/or decrease pregnancy rates. Limited studies of youth development programs also indicate that such programs may decrease adolescent pregnancy and birth rates. In addition, many AIDS education programs have greatly increased contraceptive use through increased condom use.

A review commissioned by the World Health Organization indicates that sexuality education programs "either had no effect on levels of sexual activity . . . or they delayed initiation of intercourse, and/or reduced pregnancy/abortion/birthrates in instruction recipients." Studies commissioned by the U.S. Department of Health and Human Services demonstrate that sexuality education "does not cause adolescents to initiate sex when they would not otherwise have done so."

Public Support for Sexuality Education

By a wide margin, Americans support sexuality education in schools. Eighty-two percent of American adults surveyed support requiring the provision of sexuality education in schools. When given the opportunity to remove their children from such programs, no more than one to five percent of parents actually do so. Another recent survey found that 82 percent of adults believe that educating teens about contraception is very important. Eighty-seven percent believe STD prevention education is very important. A mere 13 percent of adults believe that "teaching teenagers to abstain from sex until marriage is extremely realistic." At least 115 national organizations support comprehensive sexuality education, including: American Academy of Pediatrics, American College of Obstetricians and Gynecologists, American Medical Association, American Public Health Association,

National Education Association, National Medical Association, National School Boards Association, and Society for Adolescent Medicine.

Although abstinence-only education has garnered much recent attention, it does not address adequately the adolescent reproductive health crisis facing America's youth. By failing to provide complete and accurate information regarding contraception and STD/HIV prevention, abstinence-only sexuality education is both dangerous and counterproductive. Comprehensive sexuality education, by contrast, is an important component of a strategy to reduce unintended pregnancy, reduce the need for abortion and reduce the incidence of STDs.

"'Balanced and realistic' sexuality education programs . . . have been proven effective at delaying first intercourse and increasing use of contraception among sexually active youth."

Traditional Sex Education Can Reduce Teenage Pregnancy

Planned Parenthood Federation of America

In the following viewpoint, the Planned Parenthood Federation of America maintains that because many young people are having sex they should be informed of such consequences as pregnancy and sexually transmitted infections and how to protect themselves. Many opponents of comprehensive sex education emphasize preventing teenagers from having sex, and insist upon conveying an unquestionable message of abstinence to students. Planned Parenthood argues that this approach is unrealistic and contends that comprehensive sex education has been proven to reduce teenage pregnancy and infection. Planned Parenthood is a nonprofit organization dedicated to protecting an individual's right to make reproductive decisions and providing sexuality, reproduction, and contraceptive information and services.

As you read, consider the following questions:
1. What are three consequences of teenage pregnancy described by Planned Parenthood?
2. According to the author, what role does the media have in preventing teenage pregnancy?
3. Who does Planned Parenthood describe as high-risk teens?

Although the rate of teenage pregnancy in the United States has been declining, it remains the highest in the developed world. Approximately 97 per 1,000 women aged 15–19—one million American teenagers—become pregnant each year. The majority of these pregnancies—78 percent—are unintended.

Moreover, because the average age of menarche has reached an all-time low of about 12 or 13 years, and because four out of five young people have sex as teenagers, a greater proportion of teenage girls are at risk of becoming pregnant than ever before.

The consequences of adolescent pregnancy and childbearing are serious and numerous:

- Teen mothers are less likely to graduate from high school and more likely than their peers who delay childbearing to live in poverty and to rely on welfare.
- The children of teenage mothers are often born at low birth weight, experience health and developmental problems, and are frequently poor, abused, and/or neglected.
- Teenage pregnancy poses a substantial financial burden to society, estimated at $7 billion annually in lost tax revenues, public assistance, child health care, foster care, and involvement with the criminal justice system.

As a result, the United States needs a number of initiatives to reduce its teenage pregnancy rate and the negative outcomes that accompany it. These initiatives should incorporate medically accurate sexuality education and information in the schools and in the media, improvements in funding for and access to family planning services, and youth development programs to improve the life options of impoverished teens.

However, none of these initiatives can succeed without a general reassessment of the attitudes and mores regarding adolescent sexuality in the U.S. Presently, an unrealistic emphasis is placed on preventing adolescent sexual behavior, which overlooks the fact that sexual expression is an essential component of healthy human development for individuals of all ages. The majority of the public recognizes this fact—63 percent of Americans believe that sexual exploration among young people is a natural part of growing up. . . .

Planned Parenthood believes that policymakers must accept the fact that teens engage in sexual behavior, and they must initiate and provide funding for various programs and interventions that will facilitate responsible sexual behavior.

Medically Accurate Sexuality Education

Medically accurate sexuality education that begins in kindergarten and continues in an age-appropriate manner through the 12th grade is necessary given the early ages at which young people are initiating intercourse—7.2 percent of students nationwide report having sex before the age of 13, 42.5 percent by grade 10, and 60.9 percent by grade 12. In fact, the most successful programs aimed at reducing teenage pregnancy are those targeting younger adolescents who are not yet sexually experienced.

"Balanced and realistic" sexuality education programs that encourage students to postpone sex until they are older, but also promote safer sex practices for those who choose to become sexually active, have been proven effective at delaying first intercourse and increasing use of contraception among sexually active youth. These programs have not been shown to initiate early sexual activity or to increase levels of sexual activity or numbers of sexual partners among sexually active youth.

Sexuality education programs in the United States currently caution young people to not have sex until they are married. Of the 69 percent of school districts with a policy to teach sexuality education, 86 percent promote abstinence as the preferred or the only option for adolescents. A number of studies, however, have found that abstinence-only programs are ineffective because they fail to delay the onset of intercourse and often provide information that is medically inaccurate and potentially misleading. . . .

The vast majority of Americans support sexuality education for teenagers—93 percent believe it should be taught in high schools, and 84 percent believe it should be taught in middle or junior high schools.

Teenagers also express the need for medically accurate, responsible sexuality education:

- Nearly half of high school students nationwide report

that they need basic information on birth control, HIV/AIDS, and other sexually transmitted infections (STIs), and nearly half are unaware that having a sexually transmitted infection increases the risk of getting HIV if sexually active.

- Forty percent of students would like more information on where to get contraception; 30 percent would like more information on how to use condoms; and 51 percent would like more information on where to go to get tested for HIV and STIs.
- Forty-six percent of students do not know birth control pills can be obtained without parental permission; 21 percent do not know condoms can be purchased without parental permission; and one in five do not know free or low-cost family planning services are available for people under the age of 18. . . .

A Decline in Teenage Pregnancy

The rate of teenage pregnancy in the United States has been declining—between 1990 and 1996 it decreased from 117 pregnancies per 1,000 women aged 15–19 to 97 per 1,000, a drop of 17 percent.

A flawed report commissioned by the so-called Consortium of State Physicians Resource Councils, an anti-choice organization, concluded that the recent decline in adolescent pregnancy and childbearing is a result of higher levels of sexual abstinence among American teens. The authors attribute this increase in abstinence in part to abstinence-only education. However, this study draws its conclusions from incomplete and non-comparable data, rendering the findings invalid.

The Alan Guttmacher Institute investigated the decline in teenage pregnancy using data from the National Survey of Family Growth (NSFG), the major source of government data on population and reproductive health. The NSFG data show that the decline in teenage pregnancy rates has occurred primarily among sexually experienced teens. The fact is that sexually active teenagers are learning to use contraception more frequently and more effectively, and they account for 80 percent of the decline in teenage pregnancy rates.

The Media's Role in Pregnancy Prevention

Another source of teen information about sex is the media:

- In the U.S., one in four television programs contain a scene devoting primary emphasis to sexual behavior, and one in eight contain a scene in which intercourse is depicted or strongly implied, yet sexual precautions and the negative consequences of sexual behavior are rarely depicted.
- Research clearly shows that television portrayals contribute to sexual socialization—watching programs high in sexual content has been correlated with the early initiation of adolescent sexual intercourse.

The U.S. needs a long-term teenage pregnancy prevention media campaign that addresses the risks of sexual behavior. At present, most major networks do not air commercials or public information campaigns about sexual health. Developed countries such as the Netherlands, Germany, and France, in which teenage birth rates are four to eight times lower than that of the U.S., promote healthy, lower-risk sexual behavior through national media campaigns that have a high degree of influence with young women and men.

Teenagers Need Easy Access to Contraception

Easy and confidential access to family planning services through clinics, school-linked health centers, and condom availability programs has been found to help prevent unintended pregnancy. In 1995, contraceptive use among women aged 15–19 years old prevented an estimated 1.65 million pregnancies in the United States.

Contraceptive use is also cost-effective. The average annual cost associated with unintended pregnancy and sexually transmitted infections per adolescent who uses no method of contraception is $5,758 in the private sector and $3,079 in the public sector. Access to contraception lowers this cost. For example, the contraceptive implant costs $1,533 over five years in the private sector, saving approximately $4,225.

Various studies have demonstrated that efforts to improve teenagers' access to contraception do not increase rates of sexual activity, but do yield a number of positive outcomes.

For example:

- The most successful adolescent pregnancy prevention programs in the U.S., which combine sexuality education with direct access to or information about contraceptive services, have increased contraceptive use among participants by up to 22 percent.
- More boys who participated in a high school condom availability program in Los Angeles reported using condoms every time they engaged in vaginal intercourse during the past year (50 percent) than the year before (37 percent), and more boys reported condom use for recently initiated first vaginal intercourse (80 percent) than the year before (65 percent).
- Condom use among students in New York City public high schools that have condom availability programs is five percentage points higher than in Chicago, where no such programs exist.

Poor and Low-Income Teens

Public funding for family planning could significantly help poor (family income is at or below the federal poverty level) and low-income (family income is between 100 and 199 percent of the poverty level) teenagers aged 15–19, who account for 73 percent of young women who become pregnant, even though they make up only 38 percent of all women in that age group.

Poor teenagers are more sexually experienced than those of higher incomes, yet they use contraception less frequently and less successfully, and they have higher rates of pregnancy.

Among women aged 15–19, 60 percent of poor women are sexually experienced, versus 53 percent of low-income and 50 percent of higher income adolescents.

Nearly 60 percent of poor and low-income teenagers use some method of contraception the first time they have sex, versus 75 percent of higher income teens. Likewise, 78 percent of poor and 71 percent of low-income teenage women use contraception on an ongoing basis, versus 83 percent of higher income teens.

When faced with an unintended pregnancy, many poor and low-income teens are likely to view early childbearing as a positive, desirable choice, becoming pregnant with the misguided hope of improving their lives.

Medicaid, Title X, and the State Children's Health Insurance Program (CHIP) are three government programs that subsidize contraceptive services for poor and low-income adolescents.

Publicly funded family planning is cost-effective—every dollar spent on publicly subsidized family planning services saves $4.40 on costs that would otherwise be spent on medical care, welfare benefits, and other social services to women who became pregnant and gave birth.

Teaching Life Skills

Comprehensive sexuality education is, on the other hand, an effective strategy for giving young people the skills to delay their involvement in sexual behaviors. Several reviews of published evaluations of sexuality education, HIV prevention, and teenage pregnancy prevention programs have consistently found that:

- sexuality education does not encourage teens to start having sexual intercourse or to increase their frequency of sexual intercourse.
- programs must take place before young people begin experimenting with sexual behaviors if they are to result in a delay of sexual intercourse.
- teenagers who start having intercourse following a sexuality education program are more likely to use contraceptives than those who have not participated in a program.
- HIV programs that use cognitive and behavioral skills training with adolescents demonstrate "consistently positive" results.

Debra W. Haffner, *SIECUS*, 1997.

Of 15–19-year-olds obtaining contraceptive services, 63 percent use a publicly funded source.

Four in 10 sexually active teenagers who need contraceptive services rely upon clinics funded through Title X.

Despite these outcomes, public funding for family planning is decreasing—funding for Title X dropped 61 percent between 1980 and 1998 when inflation is taken into account. Poor teens who cannot afford the full cost of contraception must rely upon cheaper but less effective methods, such as periodic abstinence and withdrawal.

Although youth development programs for poor teens, such as academic tutoring, job training and placement, mentoring, and youth-led enterprise programs, have been found to significantly reduce teenage pregnancy rates, few adolescent pregnancy prevention programs directly address the problem of poverty.

Lesbian, bisexual, and abused teens, as well as teens who are sexually involved with older partners, are more likely than other teens to experience pregnancy, and they may need specialized programs to address their specific risk behaviors and to help them obtain services.

Pregnancy among lesbian and bisexual adolescents is 12 percent higher than among heterosexual teens. Lesbian and bisexual teens are also more likely to engage in frequent intercourse—22 percent versus 15–17 percent of heterosexual or unsure teens.

Teenagers who have been raped or abused also experience higher rates of pregnancy—in a sample of 500 teen mothers, two-thirds had histories of sexual and physical abuse, primarily by adult men averaging age 27.

Among women younger than 18, the pregnancy rate among those with a partner who is six or more years older is 3.7 times as high as the rate among those whose partner is no more than two years older. Adolescent women with older partners also use contraception less frequently—one study found that 66 percent of those with a partner six or more years older had practiced contraception at last intercourse, compared with 78 percent of those with a partner within two years of their own age.

Some states are enacting or more rigorously enforcing statutory rape laws to curb teenage pregnancy among women with older partners by deterring adult men from becoming sexually involved with minors. However, experts assert that statutory rape laws will not reduce rates of teenage pregnancy, but will discourage teens from obtaining reproductive health care out of fear that disclosing information about their partner will lead to a criminal charge.

Young men are often overlooked as a group that plays an

important role in reducing teenage pregnancy. A study of high school students in North Carolina found that 14.7 percent of sexually experienced teenage men had been involved in a pregnancy in 1997—a 38 percent increase from 1995. Sexuality educators and reproductive health care providers must therefore present pregnancy prevention as the job of both partners to foster responsible sexual choices among young men and women.

Because young men who have unprotected intercourse also tend to engage in other risk behaviors such as fighting, carrying a gun or other weapon, attempting suicide, smoking cigarettes, drinking alcohol, and using drugs, programs designed to address these behaviors should optimally include a pregnancy prevention component.

A shift in attitudes towards teenage sexuality must occur in the U.S. to facilitate the development of appropriate policies and programs to reduce teenage pregnancy. Presently, sexual activity, rather than the pregnancies that can result from it, is seen as the problem requiring intervention. Teaching young people that premarital sex is a moral failure does not prevent pregnancy—studies show that those with fearful and negative attitudes about sexuality are less likely to use contraception when they have sex than those who believe they have a right to decide to have sex.

Recognition that sexual expression is a crucial component of teenagers' development will help guarantee teenagers the right to honest, accurate information about sex and access to high quality reproductive health services that will empower them to express their sexuality in safe and healthy ways. Lower teenage pregnancy rates will follow as a natural outcome.

"The 1996 welfare reform bill is replete with language about the importance of reducing out-of-wedlock pregnancy and childbearing."

Welfare Reform May Reduce Teenage Pregnancy

Isabel V. Sawhill

The Welfare Reform Act of 1996 contains many provisions designed to reduce the number of out-of-wedlock and teenage births. Among the provisions is a requirement for minor teen mothers to live with their parents and stay in school, new funding for abstinence-only sex education in schools, and a stronger emphasis on paternity and child support obligations. In the following viewpoint, Isabel V. Sawhill argues that states have been given the tools necessary to improve present conditions, and if implemented properly, welfare reform could significantly affect the number of teen pregnancies and illegitimate births. Sawhill is a senior fellow at the Brookings Institute, a social, economic, government, and foreign policy critic.

As you read, consider the following questions:
1. According to Sawhill, what have states emphasized since the welfare reform bill instead of teenage pregnancies?
2. Why does Sawhill allege that very early childbearing, even in the context of marriage, is detrimental?
3. According to the author, how have trends in teenage sexuality changed in the 1990s?

Almost no one thinks it's a good idea for unwed teenagers to become parents. It would be the odd parent, indeed, who counseled their own teenage son or daughter to start a family, most parents hope that their children will finish school, find a job, and marry before they take on the burdens of parenthood. But what the majority of parents, almost regardless of race or social class, want for their own children is not what we have. Instead, 40 percent of all girls in the United States become pregnant before their twentieth birthday, and one out of every five goes on to become a teen mother. The overwhelming majority of these young mothers are unmarried and end up poor and on welfare.

Declining Pregnancy Rates

Certainly, recent social trends are encouraging. Teen pregnancy rates have declined—almost as sharply during the 1990s as they had increased in the preceding two decades. And for the first time, teen birth rates are dropping not because more teens are having abortions but because fewer of them are getting pregnant in the first place.

These recent declines auger well for the future, but it is worth remembering that teenage pregnancy rates in America are still at least twice as high as in other industrialized countries and about as high as they were in the early 1970s. About half of these pregnancies are carried to term while the remainder either end with a miscarriage or are terminated by an abortion. Very few teen mothers put their babies up for adoption, or marry the baby's father, a marked departure from practices 30 or 40 years ago.

When members of Congress enacted [a] new welfare law in 1996, they put at least as much emphasis on reducing teen and out-of-wedlock pregnancy as they did on requiring work. Yet states have been reluctant to take up this challenge, preferring to emphasize job placement and other strategies designed to move recipients into the workforce. In my view, that's shortsighted: Much greater attention should be given to encouraging young people to defer childbearing until they are ready to be parents. This will not be an easy task, of course. But states are now flush with funds, and some of this money ought to be invested in pregnancy-prevention programs for teenagers and in policies that re-connect fathers with their children. In the absence of such efforts, welfare reform's current success could be short-lived. If every recipient who finds a job is replaced by a younger sister ill-prepared to support a family, caseload declines will be difficult to sustain.

The strong economy has helped states to reduce welfare rolls by almost 50 percent since 1993. But the good times may not last. And when they end, it will be especially important to have in place policies that prevent young women from coming on to the rolls because of an unplanned pregnancy and birth. Even when such single parents work, they rarely have the education needed to support a family, and most will end up in low-wage, often dead-end jobs. Most of their children, whether on or off welfare, will remain poor.

Child Poverty's New Face

Poverty in the United States, especially child poverty, is increasingly associated with family structure. In the mid 1960s, when the War on Poverty began and Senator Daniel P. Moynihan, then an assistant secretary in the Department of Labor, issued his "infamous" report on illegitimacy and poverty within the black community, only 35 percent of all poor children lived in female-headed families. Today, that figure stands at almost 60 percent, and by some counts is even higher.

The proportion of all American children who are poor has been increasing from 15 percent in 1970 to 20 percent in 1996. Most of this increase is associated with the growth of single-parent families. The arithmetic behind this conclusion is straightforward. Because child poverty is five times higher in single-parent than in two-parent families, and because the proportion of all children living in fatherless families has increased dramatically, child poverty rates have increased by about five percentage points since 1970 for this reason alone.

It is not just the growth of female-headed families but also shifts in the composition of this group of single parents that have contributed to greater poverty and welfare dependency. In the 1960s and 1970s, most of the growth of single-parent families was caused by increases in divorce. In the 1980s and 1990s, all of the increase has been driven by out-of-wedlock childbearing. Currently, 32 percent of all children in the United States are born outside of marriage. The proportion is over half in many of our largest cities and close to that now in several states (e.g., Louisiana and Mississippi). Unmarried mothers tend to be younger and more disadvantaged than their divorced counterparts; as a result, they and their children are even more likely to be poor.

Finally, although out-of-wedlock childbearing is now common among women in their twenties, about half of unmarried mothers begin childbearing in their teens. So if we want to reduce such births and the poverty that accompanies them, the adolescent years are a good place to start. Not only are the consequences more dire for young girls, many of whom have not yet completed school, but these young women are less likely to marry and more likely to have additional children than those who delay parenting to a later age. The children in such families suffer the most: They are likely to have even poorer health, less success in school, and more behavioral problems than children born to older parents.

Public Policy and the Culture Wars

In the struggle against child poverty, the nation faces some difficult choices. We can make it easier for unwed mothers to raise children on their own by providing them with better education, wage supplements . . . , subsidized health insurance and child care, or other supports. Since no amount of moralizing about out-of-wedlock childbearing will change the lives of those mothers who are already struggling to raise children on their own, such aid is warranted. But looking to the future, we should encourage young people to postpone childbearing until they are married or at least prepared to support their children. Indeed, too much emphasis on supporting single-parent families at the expense of efforts to slow their growth could encourage the very trends that have left so many children in fatherless families.

The goal among those concerned about the breakdown of the family should be to discourage both too early childbearing and childbearing outside of marriage. Very early childbearing, even were it to occur within marriage, is detrimental. Such families are quite unstable, and early childbearing prevents young parents from attaining the high levels of education that are necessary to compete in today's economy. But we should also recognize that the breakdown of marriage as the normative context for raising children may have consequences for our society that are at least as profound as the age at which childbearing begins. Indeed, the teen birth rate is far lower now than it was in the 1950s. What is new is the proportion of these very early births that occur to unmarried women and the fact that single parenting has lost its stigma.

Challenging Teen Moms

[Welfare reform has] created new challenges for young mothers receiving cash assistance. Some states have implemented, along with the new eligibility requirements, services to help teenage parents respond to these challenges. These services may include special life skills training, instruction in parenting skills and pregnancy prevention, academic classes and tutoring, help in finding and paying for child care and transportation, and special attention to obtaining child support orders and support. A few states have funded group homes for teenage parents as an alternative adult-supervised living arrangement when the parental home is found to be unsafe for the young mother or her baby. In many programs, case managers work with teenage parents to identify their special needs and help arrange needed services, motivate them to comply with program requirements, and trigger changes in financial benefits (as sanctions or rewards) based on teenage parents' response.

Robert G. Wood and John Burghardt, "Implementing Welfare Reform Requirements for Teenage Parents: Lessons from Experience in Four States," October 31, 1997.

The disappearance of marriage is already far advanced in many low-income and minority communities. Liberals point to the lack of good jobs in such communities, a situation they believe has undermined the male role as bread winner. Conservatives emphasize the availability of welfare benefits, arguing that these have encouraged young women to raise children on their own. Neither explanation is strongly backed by the data, but this may be because standard social-science models cannot easily capture the dynamics of the process that has led to the breakdown of the family. For whatever reasons, monogamy is being replaced by what a team of researchers from Columbia and Princeton universities calls "fragile families." Preliminary evidence from this team's work in several cities suggests that about half of young mothers who give birth out of wedlock are cohabiting with the father of their child at the time of birth and that another 30 percent are "romantically involved." Past research suggests that such ties are not very durable, but some believe that were we to intervene at the time of the child's birth in ways that encouraged more involvement of the father it could make a difference. Offering subsidized jobs or other supports to those couples in which one parent is willing to work full-time, and both are willing to make a more durable commitment to their children, might make a difference.

In the meantime, we should emphasize reducing teen pregnancy and early childbearing, for this will surely improve the lives of children. Most early childbearing occurs outside of marriage (76 percent) and most out-of-wedlock childbearing starts in the teenage years. Divisive cultural battles about marriage will continue to lurk in the background, to be sure; but a good interim strategy that all sides should agree on is preventing early, unplanned births.

Welfare Reform to the Rescue?

The 1996 welfare reform bill is replete with language about the importance of reducing out-of-wedlock pregnancy and childbearing and restoring marriage as "the foundation of a successful society." And several of its provisions are aimed at achieving these objectives. First, the bill includes a requirement that teen mothers under the age of 18 live with their parents or in another supervised setting and remain in school. At the discretion of the state, minors can be denied all welfare benefits, an option that with a few exceptions most states have not chosen to implement. (The four that have implemented some variant of this are: Delaware, Arkansas, California, and Mississippi.)

Second, the welfare law provides an "illegitimacy bonus" to the five states with the biggest statewide drop in out-of-wedlock childbearing among all women, not just those on welfare or those who are teenagers. The drop must be accomplished without any increase in abortion. The first bonuses, totalling $20 million per state, were awarded in the fall of 1999 to Alabama, California, the District of Columbia, Massachusetts, and Michigan, based on drops experienced from 1994–95 to 1996–97. Third, the bill provides new funding of $50 million a year for abstinence education programs to states willing to match every four dollars of federal funds with three dollars of state funds. The bill stipulates that the monies only be used for programs that advocate abstinence until marriage and do not teach about contraception.

Fourth, the bill emphasizes establishing paternity and enforcing the child-support obligations of absent parents. To that end, it requires employers to report all new hires to the child-support enforcement authorities for purposes of tracking down delinquent fathers. And other features of the bill call upon states to more vigorously enforce statutory rape laws and the Department of Health and Human Services to develop a strategy for preventing out-of-wedlock teen pregnancies. Health Education Services (HES) is also charged with ensuring that 25 percent of all communities in the United States have a pregnancy-prevention program for teenagers. (No funds were provided for this purpose, but HES claims that 30 percent of all communities have programs that meet the requirements of the law.)

Finally, the bill gives states great discretion in how they use their welfare monies, as long as they achieve the basic purposes of the Welfare Reform Act. For example, states are allowed to use the funds for teen-pregnancy prevention, family planning for those already on welfare, fatherhood programs, and other activities that might reduce teen-pregnancy and out-of-wedlock childbearing. The bill also permits states to impose a "family cap" (denial of benefits for children born or conceived while their mother is on welfare). Twenty-one states have chosen to impose such a cap (and two others provide flat grants, regardless of family size).

Overall, it is hard to argue that states have not been given most of the tools and incentives they need to reduce out-of-wedlock and teenage childbearing. I say most because the one area where states are still constrained, or have constrained themselves, is with respect to abortion. In addition, one of the bill's provisions—the abstinence money—has been highly controversial with some reproductive-rights groups, which have urged states not to apply for the funds. But in the end, all states did. States also have the resources to tackle the problem of teenage childbearing. As of early 1999, they had $4.2 billion in unspent and uncommitted welfare funds, according to the Department of Health and Human Services, that could be devoted to this and other purposes (assuming Congress doesn't permanently rescind the money).

It is true that most pregnancy-prevention programs for teenagers have been inadequately evaluated and that there are no sure-fire solutions to the problem. However, many promising models have been identified. The best sex-education programs are comprehensive in coverage and factually accurate, though they are not necessarily "value-free." Indeed, they take a clear stance on the behaviors in question. They teach teenagers not just the facts of life but, more importantly, how to resist peer pressure. Other effective approaches include after-school programs, mentoring, and community service, all of which provide alternatives to early sex and pregnancy. . . .

How Social Norms Work

Prior to 1990, teen pregnancy rates had been creeping up for two decades. Although sex education in the schools and family-planning services expanded, so did the proportion of teens having sex. And in this battle between sex and safe sex, sex won. At the same time that technology was making it easier to prevent pregnancy, social norms that had once condemned sex outside of marriage became far more permissive. Focus-group interviews with today's teenagers indicate that sex during the teen years is widely accepted. A 1997 study from Child Trends reports that boys in particular are teased or taunted if they are not sexually active while those who have multiple partners often gain in reputation. Although girls who resist sex are not ostracized, they are subject to subtle pressures from boys; often girls will have sex to secure or maintain a relationship. These pressures from peers are rein-forced by the popular media, which glamorize sex, and by adults who are ambivalent about their own values or insuffi-ciently involved in their teenagers' lives. The result is that by the mid 1990s, a high proportion of teenagers were sexually experienced—about one-fifth by the age of 15 and three-fifths by the age of 18. At the same time, women were mar-rying later, creating a longer period during which nonmarital births could occur. (Girls in the United States typically reach puberty at age 12 or 13 but don't marry until age 25.)

Not only were teens initiating sex earlier, but in addition, sex education and access to family-planning clinics were no panacea. Sex education is now available in over 90 percent of high schools, and most teenagers are fully informed about how pregnancies occur, but sex-education courses often are too short and come too late to do much good. In addition, the controversies and sensitivities surrounding them have prevented public school teachers from providing the kind of guidance they might give their own children at home. And although contraceptives are widely available, not just in clin-ics but also in stores, and teens are using them much more frequently than in the past, they do not use them consis-tently. The result is that failure rates are high and unplanned pregnancies all too common. Consider, for example, the 15 percent annual failure rate for those relying on condoms, the most prevalent form of contraception among teens: At this rate, more than half of sexually active individuals will be-come pregnant within five years and if, as we suspect, teens are especially poor users of contraceptives, the number could be far higher.

The good news of the 1990s is that sexual activity has de-clined at the same time that contraceptive use has continued to increase. No one knows why we have had this double dose of good news in the 1990s. But social norms seem to be shifting in a more conservative direction. For example, ac-cording to one study, the proportion of college freshmen who believe "it's all right for two people to have sex even if they've known each other for a very short time" dropped from 52 percent in 1987 to 42 percent in 1997. Similarly, the Urban Institute analysis found that two-thirds of the drop in sexual activity among adolescent males since 1988 was directly attributable to a shift in their attitudes. This shift may have been prompted by the prevalence of AIDS and other sexually transmitted diseases that are rampant among teens. Other factors may have included welfare reform, a strong economy, and a variety of private as well as governmental efforts to educate the public about the risks of casual sex. . . .

A Return of Victorian Values?

We could be on the cusp of a new social trend. Although the data are still fragmentary and the thesis must remain tentative, it appears that sexual attitudes are becoming more conservative and that both safer sex and delayed sex are gaining ground. Teen pregnancy and birth rates have declined for most of the decade and the out-of-wedlock birth ratio has stabilized.

Those looking for guaranteed, programmatic solutions to the problems of teen pregnancy and out-of-wedlock births are likely to be disappointed, however. The point is not that programs can't be effective, but that without a change in social norms, their impact may be small. Conversely, an intervention that begins by affecting behavior in quite modest ways may eventually produce changes in norms that snowball into bigger long-term effects. Teenagers, in particular, are enormously influenced by what their friends, parents, and heroes say and do. This suggests that programs not be judged only on the basis of their immediate effects but also on their potential to reorient peer culture. It also suggests that devoting funds to media campaigns and supporting faith-based or local community efforts that put values before services would be effective.

The subtler point is that services and values cannot be delivered in isolation from one another. Sex-education programs that teach adolescents about their bodies but not how to deal with their feelings for one another and the values that should guide such relationships are likely to fail. Similarly, "just say no" campaigns that don't engage young people in constructive activities and connect them to a supportive peer group and community are also likely to be a waste of time.

In sum, reducing births to unwed teenagers could substantially decrease child poverty, welfare dependency, and other social ills. Although little is known with certainty about how to advance this objective, states working in partnership with civic and faith-based institutions now have the opportunity to experiment with a variety of promising approaches that are critical to the longer-term success of current welfare reform efforts.

> *"Just as the current welfare system rewards failure rather than progress, it creates a set of perverse incentives and harmful expectations for many teens."*

Welfare Benefits Do Not Reduce Teenage Pregnancy

Kathleen Sylvester

In the following viewpoint, Kathleen Sylvester argues that the current welfare system has had detrimental effects on the family by "normalizing" the unfortunate circumstance of single parenthood and, most often, motherhood. Statistics prove that children of teenage parents often have children as teenagers themselves, perform poorly in school, and end up on welfare. To reverse this destructive trend she contends that the welfare system must be restructured and made less appealing to teenagers and potential parents. Sylvester is the director of the Social Policy Action Network, which promotes effective social policy by transforming the ideas and findings of front-line practitioners into concrete action agendas for policymakers.

As you read, consider the following questions:
1. Briefly explain the pattern of life for a pregnant teenager, as described by Sylvester.
2. What are two reasons the author offers for teenage girls choosing to have children?
3. What were the purposes of the original neighborhood opportunity centers, according to Sylvester?

All across America, young girls who still are children themselves are bearing children of their own. It is a calamity for these young mothers, because early motherhood denies them opportunities and choices; for their offspring, because most will grow up poor and without a father; and for the nation, because these youngsters are likely to repeat the tragic cycle of poverty and dysfunction into which they were born. However, it is a calamity that is preventable.

Compelling evidence now supports what most Americans long have understood intuitively. Family structure and lifestyle, as well as economics, influence how children turn out. Those of young, unmarried mothers fare badly, and society pays the cost. The equation is straightforward: As poverty is the most accurate predictor of teen pregnancy, teen pregnancy is a near certain predictor of poverty. Two-thirds of never married mothers raise their kids in poverty.

Children of unmarried teen mothers are far more likely than those of older, two parent families to fall behind and drop out of school, get into trouble with the law, abuse drugs and join gangs, have children of their own out of wedlock, and become dependent on welfare.

The situation is urgent. There are over 9,000,000 youngsters living in welfare families. As they reach adolescence, many are "scripted" to repeat the lives of their parents. It is vital to intervene and break the cycle before those children, too, become parents too soon and create a new generation of disadvantage.

To reverse this cycle requires a categorical declaration by civic, moral, and community leaders that it is wrong—not simply foolish or impractical—for women and men to make babies they can not support emotionally and financially. It also is time to challenge the complacent view that having babies out of wedlock is simply a lifestyle choice, and that since all such preferences are equally valid, no behavior should be condemned. This stance is untenable in the face of compelling evidence that not all choices are equal in terms of their impact on youngsters, and that children need fathers as well as mothers. . . .

The pattern of life for a poor young woman who becomes pregnant and has a child is predictable. She is likely to have one more child—usually within two years. If she has a second child, she is less likely to finish high school, unlikely to marry and is at great risk of cycling in and out of the welfare system for a significant portion of her life.

The social costs for offspring of teen mothers also are apparent. Compared to those living in two-parent families, children in single-parent households score worse on measures of health, education, and emotional and behavioral adjustment. Later on, if they continue to live with never-married single parents, they become more likely to drop out of school, become heads of single-parent families themselves and experience a lower socioeconomic status as adults.

Youngsters who grow up in single-parent households are at much greater risk of drug and alcohol abuse, mental illness, suicide, poor educational performance, and criminality, according to the National Commission on Children. Two-thirds of the occupants of juvenile detention centers are young men who grew up without fathers, many of whom already have sired children who will grow up without fathers as well. Such consequences are not hard to comprehend. It is difficult to socialize the next generation in neighborhoods where a new generation is born every 14 years.

The Costs to Society

Any public campaign against teen pregnancy should emphasize how costly it is for all citizens to ignore the situation. The Center for Population Options estimates that 53% of outlays for Aid to Families with Dependent Children (AFDC), food stamps and Medicaid are attributable to households begun by teen births. Medical services for teen mothers and their kids are especially costly. Young, poor, unmarried, uneducated, and uninsured mothers are much less likely than older, more stable mothers to obtain prenatal care. Pregnant teens frequently deny their pregnancies in the early stages and have poor access to medical services.

Infants born to younger women are more likely to be born prematurely, die in the neonatal period, and be of low birth weight. Each low-birth weight baby averages $20,000 in hospital costs; total lifetime medical expenses for such children can average $400,000.

One in four sexually active teens contracts at least one sexually transmitted disease, posing serious health risks to mothers and their offspring. Because large numbers have sex without adequate protection and many have multiple partners, teens are a very high-risk group. As a social worker at a clinic in Maryland explained, once any sexually transmitted disease is introduced into a group of sexually active teens, it can spread exponentially.

The Welfare System

The social welfare system—created to help single mothers because society recognized that families without a father's presence were disadvantaged—has created an unintended consequence. It has "normalized" single-parent families. The dilemma is this: Everything the welfare system does to create normal and acceptable lives for the children of teen mothers leads to the perception that their parents' behavior is normal and acceptable.

Just as the current welfare system rewards failure rather than progress, it creates a set of perverse incentives and harmful expectations for many teens. When a young woman who is poor has a child out of wedlock, the social welfare bureaucracy offers her financial support, special attention, and some measure of independence. She receives more attention by having a baby than a young woman who delays childbearing.

The system marginalizes fathers by replacing them with welfare checks. Jobless young men often are shunned by the families of their girlfriends and dismissed by the social welfare establishment as useless or a bad influence on their own children. The system discounts their non-monetary value to their offspring—their potential to help nurture and care for those kids.

In many communities, young men and women grow up in families where females are viewed as self-sufficient and males as unnecessary. If families appear to be functioning without fathers, why should young women seek fathers for their children? Why should men feel compelled to take responsibility for them?

The welfare system is just one factor in the set of decisions that leads to early childbearing. For many teens, having a baby fulfills needs for intimacy, independence, and peer approval. . . .

Reasons for Teenage Parenthood

In recent years, two more disturbing factors about young men's motivations have emerged. Ronald Mincy [editor of *Nurturing Young Black Males,*] cites the lack of responsible male role models in underclass communities. Since the mid 1970s, the decline in demand for low-skill jobs has undermined the economic status of African-American fathers who lack a college degree. The position of working-class males in black communities—individuals who once served as important socializing agents, especially for boys and young men—has been eroded by glossier, higher-profile gang members and hustlers. In addition, young men who live in violent urban neighborhoods sometimes view paternity as a means of "replacing themselves" before they die. Most of teenage male deaths are attributable to the use of guns.

The reasons that young women choose to bear children are even more complicated. For many teenagers, pregnancy may not be a conscious choice. Johns Hopkins University researcher Laurie Schwab Zabin, who studied young women taking pregnancy tests in Baltimore, reported that less than five percent said they had planned to become pregnant, while nearly half expressed negative feelings and the other half "ambivalence" about sex, contraception, and pregnancy. According to the National Survey of Families and Households, 15% of births to teens are described by mothers 17 and younger as being wanted at the time, compared with 33% of births to 18- and 19-year-olds.

There is a growing body of research to explain this behavior. Most teen mothers are daughters of teen mothers, and many are daughters of women who suffer from periods of depression and who left their own mothers' homes while their children still were very young. With no father or grandparents to turn to, a young woman whose main source of emotional support is a single mother, poorly equipped to be a good nurturer, may seek emotional attachment by becoming sexually active or by having a child of her own.

The pattern among teen parents is fairly consistent. After the birth of a baby—or frequently even before it—the father has moved on in search of another conquest. As the responsibility for the child falls to the young mother, she becomes disillusioned with male intimacy. The new mother discovers, however, that there are advantages to having a baby, and her family often accepts responsibility for the child. Research shows that, at this point in the decision-making process, teens' assessments are deeply affected by their families. Grandmothers, who frequently were teen mothers themselves, often eagerly assume primary responsibility for grandchildren in what they view as a second chance at motherhood.

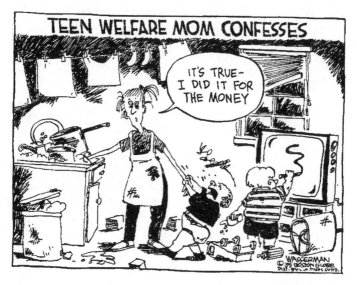

Wasserman. © 1995 by *Boston Globe*. Reprinted by permission of Los Angeles Times Syndicate.

A baby also provides status. The state officially recognizes and provides assistance to a young woman with a child. Moreover, she now has ammunition in the status battles that occur between teen mothers in the inner city: whose baby is cuter and whose is better dressed? Young mothers form a community with common interests and develop stronger bonds than they had before their children were born.

Finally, for many young women, a child is an economic asset. A baby and the ensuing support of the welfare system—with its guaranteed income and medical care, food stamps, and subsidized housing—may seem the surest way to make a life. In this context, childbearing is not a wholly unreasonable decision in the short term.

Changing the Rules of Welfare

To make teenage parenting less attractive for both young women and men, the first step is changing the rules of the welfare game. There must be obvious and immediate negative consequences for choosing unmarried parenting. Young women who are minors no longer should be allowed to set up independent households. School-age mothers must stay in school or participate in job training. Young men as well as young women must be held accountable for their actions with requirements to stay in school, work, or make in-kind contributions to the welfare of their children. . . .

In implementing such requirements, there must be a series of changes in the welfare environment that make it possible to hold them to these new standards. The notion of requiring mothers under age 18 to live with a parent sounds like a practical and reasonable solution. In many cases, it is not. The mothers of these young women frequently are lacking in parenting skills themselves. Many teens, moreover, come from homes where they have been subjected to sexual or physical abuse. That is why it is necessary to construct a new environment. Young women must be offered stable and safe places to raise their children.

Second-Chance Homes

The first building block of this new environment should be a national network of "second-chance homes." Teen welfare mothers who are judged to come from unstable or unsafe households would be required to live in these homes as a condition for receiving welfare. In earlier eras, homes for unwed mothers offered shelter and support to pregnant teens before their babies were born. As out-of-wedlock childbearing was destigmatized, most of them disappeared. Now that many young women are choosing to keep their babies, it is time to bring these homes back in a new form.

Introducing community-based second chance homes, supervised by older couples, could offer young mothers a refuge from the difficulties of their own families. They also would provide them with an opportunity to observe a respectful and caring relationship between a woman and a man, and to expose their young kids to a responsible male role model.

At the same time, the homes would provide the structure and discipline these young mothers will need to satisfy the obligations they must meet in order to receive welfare payments. When teen mothers are required to return to school, they will have reliable day care. When they are required to take parenting classes, they will have support in practicing what they have been taught. Teen mothers often are eager to learn about child development and nutrition, but have no one to teach them. In other instances, they acquire practical child-rearing skills in parenting classes, but face opposition from their own mothers, whose child-rearing practices were different. . . .

Neighborhood Opportunity Centers

The next step in changing the welfare culture is offering welfare recipients opportunities to improve their own lives and that of their communities. A national network of neighborhood opportunity centers would expand informal networks of social support and allow families to help each other.

The idea is not new. It grows out of the experience of the settlement houses that helped European immigrants assimilate into America nearly a century ago. The settlement houses did not define disadvantaged citizens in terms of dysfunction; rather, they emphasized social activities that brought people together and capitalized on their strengths. Most were privately funded and reflected community consensus about what role they should play in helping families.

A handful of these institutions remain active in communities across the country. They offer "resource exchanges" where neighbors can make "deposits" by contributing services and "withdrawals" for services they need. Those unable to make deposits can draw upon balances accrued by volunteers. Members exchange babysitting, transportation assistance, and home repair help. Some centers offer summer camps, exercise classes, and adult education. They sponsor homework clubs for schoolchildren and friendship groups for people of all ages.

This concept should be revived and used as a model for a national network of neighborhood opportunity centers. These need not be new, bureaucratic, government-run institutions. Every community has schools or centers attached to schools that could be the focal point for offering families opportunities to connect with one another and with resources in their own communities.

These centers can strengthen supports that help families deal with stress, reduce isolation, and have a positive effect on families by recognizing that they have "assets" to offer their communities. Such positive experiences are known to improve "mothers'" perceptions of themselves and their kids; fathers' involvement in childrearing; children's self-esteem; and youngsters' school success. . . .

Third, every welfare family should receive a "passport" out of welfare. With welfare reform's strong emphasis on reciprocity and entry into the workplace, it is sensible to link those two ideas together. That means defining work broadly and giving welfare recipients credit for productive activities that lead them back to work.

Reciprocity should begin as soon as a welfare recipient starts receiving benefits. Every welfare family should get a passport, designed like the "smart cards" used for banking. Every member of the family could earn credit toward satisfying requirements for the monthly welfare check. Such a system would be based on the idea that everyone on welfare can and should be actively engaged in a productive lifestyle. . . .

The Separation of Sex and Marriage

The sexual revolution, the development of effective contraceptives, and legalized abortion have contributed to a "delinking" of sex and marriage. As a healthier U.S. population matures sexually at an earlier age, yet does not mature emotionally any sooner, a growing biological gap emerges between the onset of puberty and the ability to manage its consequences.

A changing economy and changing marriage patterns have created a similar gap. A high school education no longer equips a young man or woman with skills that can support a family. Thus, most young people delay marriage—but not sexual activity—until their mid 20s.

Sensible policy must take these changes into account. Society must stop condemning all sexual activity by all teenagers and redefine "moral behavior" as responsible sexual activity. The crucial distinction between sexual behavior and the socially undesirable outcomes of sexual behavior must be acknowledged. It must be reasserted that children belong inside marriage.

Two messages must be conveyed to young people simultaneously. First, the younger teens should abstain from sex until they are mature enough to understand the consequences of their actions and make informed decisions. Second, when teens are old enough to make that choice, they must do so responsibly. They must not endanger their own health and the health of their partners with unprotected sex, unwanted pregnancies, or unnecessary abortions.

The conflict over what young people should be taught about sex and what values that teaching imparts in many instances has led to paralysis. In the debate over whether abstinence or contraception is the right message, often neither is offered. . . .

There is no instant solution that will reduce the 80–90% teenage pregnancy rates in America's inner cities overnight. A social change that took decades to become a crisis can not be eradicated in a year or two. However, the trend can—and must—be reversed.

"Leaving males out of the equation clearly limits the effectiveness of teen pregnancy prevention efforts."

Male Involvement Programs Can Reduce Teenage Pregnancy

Kristin A. Moore, Anne K. Driscoll, and Theodora Ooms

Most teenage pregnancy prevention programs focus on young girls, because they bear the consequences of unintended pregnancies. In the following viewpoint, Kristin A. Moore, Anne K. Driscoll, and Theodora Ooms argue that more emphasis should be placed on educating young men and boys on contraception, safe sex, and responsibility. She contends that society is increasingly holding young men responsible for illegitimate children by enacting stricter child support regulations, and boys need to be taught not only how to act responsibly, but also to take responsibility for careless actions. Moore, Driscoll, and Ooms are affiliated with Child Trends, a non-profit research organization.

As you read, consider the following questions:

1. As quoted by the author, what does William Marsiglio call three types of procreators?
2. What are three activities Ooms describes of male involvement programs?
3. According to the author, what is the difference between maleness and manhood?

Everyone knows that it takes two to create a pregnancy, but, until recently, efforts to reduce teen pregnancy often left boys and young men out of the picture. To understand more about this omission and new efforts to remedy it, the National Campaign to Prevent Teen Pregnancy and the Family Impact Seminar co-sponsored a roundtable meeting of scholars, practitioners, policy officials, and representatives from organizations serving male youth. The purpose was to review research about male sexual behavior, to get the facts straight about the age differences between teen girls and their male partners, and to explore the lessons being learned from the growing number of efforts to target males in teen pregnancy prevention. This report is based primarily on a background paper for the meeting, panel presentations at the meeting itself, and general roundtable discussions.

Key Facts About Male Sexual Behavior

Sexual Activity. Throughout the 1970s and 1980s, the percentage of all teenagers engaging in sexual intercourse steadily increased. However, there is some evidence that teen sexual activity may have leveled off in recent years. With regard to males, in 1988, 60 percent of never-married males aged 15–19 reported having had sex. By 1995, only 55 percent of never-married males aged 15–19 reported having had sexual intercourse.

Contraception. Although reported condom use at first intercourse by males aged 15–19 increased substantially from 55 percent in 1988 to 69 percent in 1995, many young men still do not use contraceptives consistently, placing them at risk of creating a pregnancy.

Risk of Causing an Out-of-Wedlock Pregnancy. With the average age of first marriage for males at 26 years, many young men typically have long periods of sexual activity before marriage. The average gap between first intercourse and marriage for young men is ten years, a period during which many males are at risk of making a girl or young woman pregnant. This gap is especially wide for African-American males (about 19 years) and somewhat narrower for Hispanics, who are more likely to marry in their teen years.

Responsible Attitudes. While many young men often engage in behaviors that put them at risk of making teen girls pregnant, most hold responsible attitudes about pregnancy prevention and parenting, according to the National Survey of Adolescent Men. More than 90 percent agreed that one should not have sex without contraception, that sexual partners should discuss contraception, and that males should be responsible for children that they bring into the world. . . .

Understanding Male Sexual Development and Behavior

To help boys and young men avoid causing teen pregnancies, one needs a sound understanding of the developmental stages and factors influencing male sexual behavior. Researchers at the roundtable meeting described how biology, psychology, relations with family and peers, the broader culture, and institutions like schools and the media all influence young men's sexual attitudes and actions. Cultural messages about sexuality, sexual behavior, and becoming parents—as well as access to reproductive health services—also affect young men's sexual conduct. They mature at different rates than young women, and society has different expectations regarding their behavior. Pregnancy prevention initiatives must be tailored according to these differences.

Adolescence presents boys with a particular set of tasks and challenges. Throughout their teenage years, young men are developing a sense of their identity—in terms of gender (what does it mean to be a man?), vocation (what skills do I have? what work can I do?), and relationships (whom will I love? who are my friends?). They strive for autonomy and independence, yet need also to stay connected with their families. They learn more abstract modes of thinking and reasoning and gradually develop the ability to weigh present gains against future costs.

Young men who impregnate teen girls come in a variety of forms, according to sociologists. In panelist William Marsiglio's terminology, a few "naive procreators" may be unaware of the consequences of having sex, but, more often, teen males are "careless procreators," more interested in "scoring" than worried about the consequences. Some young men are "deliberate procreators" because they see paternity as a source of prestige and as a way of affirming their manhood.

Stages of Male Adolescent Development

Experts emphasize the importance of distinguishing among early, middle, and late adolescence. Early adolescent males, around 12 to 14 years of age, are just beginning to show the physical signs of sexual maturity. Some experiment sexually, but they are unlikely to get a girl pregnant because of underdeveloped sperm production, among other reasons. However, this does not mean they are incapable of causing a pregnancy. While early adolescence is an opportune time to encourage delay in sexual activity, the typical 12-year-old is concrete and short-term in his thinking. Arguments about long-term benefits or harm are unlikely to be effective; rather, boys this age are more responsive to positive feedback from caring adults.

The typical middle adolescent, aged 15 to 17, challenges limits and authority as he experiments with new ways of behaving. He believes that no serious harm can befall him. This sense of invulnerability enables teens to move away from family and become more independent, but also may lead them to take unnecessary risks. Fifteen-to 17-year-old boys are not motivated by scare tactics. Their self-esteem depends largely on the views of their peers. They may engage in peer-bonding activities focused on sex, such as having locker room discussions and reading or viewing adult sexual material. Intervention programs focused on changing group social norms are often most effective.

Adolescents who are 17 years old and older are sexually mature but typically are still struggling to develop their identities. A young man of this age often acts with exaggerated bravado in his relationships with young women. In today's society, because many boys grow up without a strong, consistent relationship with a father or father figure, it is much harder for them to learn what it is to be a responsible man. That is why involving grown men in prevention initiatives is critical. And for boys and young men in communities where jobs are scarce, violence is endemic, and incarceration common, aggression and violence may seem manly and danger exciting; a certain callousness toward women may also develop. Programs must deal with such complex issues and not just address sexual behavior in isolation.

Although we know quite a bit about the psycho-social-sexual development of young males, there is still a lot to learn. Too often, we study only youths who get in trouble. We must also study the many teen males (and females) who manage to avoid high-risk behaviors and abstain from sexual intercourse or unprotected sex, drinking, and drugs. Research also focuses too much on individual behavior; we must conduct research on the relationships between couples—how they communicate about sex and other aspects of their relationships. Finally, we need to learn more about how the media—and other aspects of the environment boys grow up in—affects their sexual attitudes and behavior.

What Are Male Involvement Programs?

Traditionally, school-based pregnancy prevention programs have included teen males, but—since females clearly have more at stake—the primary purpose of the curricula has been to affect the attitudes and behaviors of and choices made by teen girls. Prevention efforts sponsored by family planning clinics and health centers have for the most part been designed for women, as well.

Public policy is increasingly holding males financially responsible for the children they father outside of marriage—witness, for example, the strict child support enforcement provisions of the recent federal welfare reform. For the same reasons, boys and men must also be held accountable for teen pregnancy. Leaving males out of the equation clearly limits the effectiveness of teen pregnancy prevention efforts. Thus, there is growing interest in understanding the male role in teen pregnancy and in finding effective ways of explicitly targeting men and boys in prevention initiatives.

Over the past decade, and especially within the last three years, a growing number of exciting and innovative programs and initiatives have been designed to help boys and young men avoid causing teen pregnancy. Most are community-based, but a few are state-wide or national in scope. They are a varied lot with different goals and philosophies. The community-based programs take place in different settings, under different sponsors, and target different ages and populations of males. Some reach out to boys in school, while others focus on those in juvenile detention settings or on fathers whose children are in Head Start [an organization that provides support for low-income families with young children]. Some train health care providers who work with young men. Others work with male youths in recreation and sports settings. Some programs are free-standing; others are part of a larger program providing a variety of services to young men. Some are staffed primarily by men, including volunteers from the community. Others are staffed by health educators, who may be women or men. While most of these programs seek to tailor their messages specifically to males and most of their activities are for males only, a few also include activities designed to bring the two sexes together to talk about their relationships.

The Crucial Role of Males

Why males were ever excluded from the way we think about pregnancy prevention is puzzling. Sexual behavior involves two partners, and decisions to have sex and to use contraception undoubtedly reflect both partners' perspectives, whether explicitly or implicitly. Yet fertility and family are traditionally ascribed to the world of females—a perspective that has kept us from acknowledging what should have been obvious—that males must be involved in any policy solution to unintended pregnancies among teenagers.

It is well known, for instance, that adolescent boys initiate sex earlier than girls and that they tend to accumulate more sexual partners over their lifetimes. Even though males do not actually get pregnant, it does not make sense to segregate them from prevention efforts when they have sex earlier, more frequently, and with more partners than females of comparable ages.

Freya L. Sonenstein et al., "Involving Males in Preventing Teen Pregnancy: A Guide for Program Planners," January 1998.

Most of these programs try to affect motivation, change attitudes, and develop the skills needed for boys and young men to act responsibly in their relations with teen girls. Some are specifically focused on sex-related behavior and responsibilities; others aim to help young men consider broader values, hopes, and ideals (for example, what it means to be a man and a father). Most promote sexual abstinence, especially for younger teens. Some programs promote abstinence until marriage and encourage those who have been sexually active to become secondary or "born-again" virgins. Others, assuming that most older teen boys and young men will be sexually active, offer information about contraception.

Program activities vary—media campaigns employing posters and public service announcements that promote male responsibility; magazines aimed specifically at young boys; peer information, education, and support groups; one-on-one mentoring; and counseling. While growing in number, male involvement programs are still few, and their funding base is fragile and short-term. Few have existed for more than two to three years, and no evaluations are yet available assessing their impact on reducing teen pregnancy. Questions remain about how to replicate and institutionalize these programs over the long haul. . . .

Structuring Male Involvement Programs

Despite the diversity among the various programs, there was a striking consensus among roundtable participants on the broad principles that should guide the structure, design, and overall messages of pregnancy prevention initiatives designed for boys and young men.

Make the Male Focus Mainstream. Teen pregnancy prevention initiatives must incorporate a male perspective throughout their programming. Boys and young men respond to different messages and approaches than do girls and young women. Thus, some messages should be designed specifically for boys and men, and some activities should be offered separately to males. A focus on boys and men in teen pregnancy prevention must become mainstream, not just an occasional, add-on component with little or no connection to the larger initiatives.

Tailored Approaches. Male involvement initiatives must tailor their efforts to their audiences' particular ages and stages of development. For example, because 15- and 16-year-old boys believe themselves to be invulnerable and are inveterate risk-takers, scare tactics about the risks of STDs or pregnancy will not motivate them in the same way that such tactics might influence older teens or young men.

Look for Male Youth Where They Are. Prevention efforts should reach out to boys and men in community settings where they naturally congregate, through the media channels they tune to, and at times when they are available. School-based efforts are clearly insufficient by themselves because male school dropouts are at high risk of engaging in unprotected sexual activity and young adult men are often the sexual partners of teenage women.

Establishing Trust

Males Need a "Safe" Place. Male-only activities create an atmosphere of trust—a "safe" place where boys and young men can reveal their hopes, worries, fears, and ignorance about sexuality and male-female relationships to older adult men and to their peers. However, some believe it can also be useful to bring young males and females together to talk about these issues.

Use Adult Males as Mentors and Role Models. Many teen boys and young men, especially from communities at high risk of teen pregnancy, lack positive relationships with their fathers and other older males who can serve as responsible role models and mentors. Successful male involvement programs involve male program staff, as well as adult males from the community, in designing and implementing activities. Some experience suggests that while older adults may successfully lead programs and craft messages, the most effective people to deliver messages to teen men are their slightly older peers—that is, males five to seven years older. The relationships between the young men served and the program staff and volunteers are critical in assuring the continued participation of the teens.

Understand and Build on the Participants' Cultural and Religious Backgrounds. Male involvement programs are most effective when they respect the cultural, racial, and religious backgrounds of the participants. In first-generation immigrant communities, for example, one needs to understand the cultural values of the nations from which the young men have come. For example, Los Compadres, a program in Santa Barbara, California, helps Latino youth rediscover the original meaning of "machismo"—that is, the responsibility of being a man—and the Rites of Passage Collective in Baltimore, which serves African-American youth, draws upon African concepts of social hierarchy and respect for elders to create rituals of manhood development.

Embed the Program in the Community. Successful programs consult extensively with community members from the first stages of planning to get input on goals and activities and to allay concerns. This is particularly important in communities beset by violence and racism, where youth often develop a sense of fatalism that makes planning for a pregnancy-free adolescence difficult and where trust in public institutions may be low. For instance, community involvement is a major focus of the St. Thomas Plain Talk Project in New Orleans. This consultative process, which needs to be ongoing, can help bring in new insights and valuable resources. Community involvement and support also helps ensure program longevity.

Communicating Clearly

Engage in "Plain Talk." Information should be presented in clear, concise, and concrete terms, free of technical or scientific jargon. For example, instead of saying "Fifty percent of your friends will make a girl pregnant before they are 20," point to three young men in a group of six.

Craft Positive, Male-Friendly Messages. Some earlier efforts to target boys and men in teen pregnancy prevention used scare tactics and messages that blamed their target audiences. Program leaders are now convinced that these approaches don't work and just make young men defensive. Messages that appeal to hopes and dreams seem to work better—for example, "Be Proud, Be Responsible, Be a Man" from California's Men Do Care program, "Show Your True Strength;" used in Austin, Texas, and "True Love Waits;" a program developed by the National Federation for Catholic Youth Ministry.

Emphasize the Difference Between Maleness and Manhood. Unfortunately, teen boys and young men have learned from the media and their peers that being a "real man" means being aggressive, "scoring" with as many women as possible, and, for some, getting a woman pregnant. In contrast, many male involvement programs work hard to help youth redefine their understanding of "manhood" and to emphasize caring, responsibility, commitment to family, self-control, and greater respect for women. Some programs create special rituals that serve as "rites of passage" to manhood. Many abstinence-based programs emphasize the rewards of remaining celibate until marriage.

Connect Sexuality with Procreation. Since most young women think about themselves as potential mothers, they usually connect having sex with the risk of pregnancy. Studies have shown that young men are much less likely to connect sexual activity with the possibility of becoming a father. Some male involvement programs try to make that connection by helping teen boys reflect on what their experience of fatherhood has been, think about when they will be ready to be a father, and imagine what kind of father they will want to be.

Different Points of View

On some issues, however, there is less consensus among those working in male involvement initiatives. For example, some believe only men can effectively reach boys and young men. Others feel that women can do so just as well. Some strongly recommend adopting holistic approaches that view sex in the context of a youth's overall development and, thus, design efforts to prevent a range of high-risk behaviors, including sex, drinking, and drug use. Others feel strongly that sexuality, which is in itself normal and good, should not be equated with drug and alcohol abuse, which are harmful. They recommend focusing solely on promoting responsible sexual behavior. . . .

One group of initiatives targeting young men strongly promotes the goal of sexual abstinence until marriage. Proponents maintain this avoids the inconsistency of a message that says "Be abstinent, but if you are going to have sex, use contraception." They urge youth to understand that abstinence is the only 100-percent effective way of avoiding pregnancy and STDs, and that many youth suffer emotionally from casual and brief sexual relationships. Abstinence advocates say they have found that young men respond favorably to research suggesting that there may be tangible rewards to waiting until marriage (such as better sex within marriage and more stable marriages). Proponents of this point of view believe that teenagers are frequently "undersold," that they can and do respond to higher moral standards. Also, they argue that it is a mistake to assume that if a teen has had sex once, there is no going back. Many teens can resume an abstinent lifestyle.

Another group of male involvement initiatives promotes abstinence for younger boys and protected sex for sexually active boys and young men. These programs assume that nonmarital sex is not invariably wrong, as long as contraceptives are used, pregnancy and disease are avoided, and mutual commitment, consent, and caring are present. These "abstinence plus" proponents point out that premarital sex has existed throughout history but that in the past couples were pressured to get married when the young women got pregnant. Now out-of-wedlock childbearing is not stigmatized, and, as a consequence, more than three-quarters of teen births occur outside of marriage (compared to 15 percent in 1960). Moreover, there are some communities in which jobs are scarce, and wages are too low to support a family. In these communities, in particular, men marry much later or do not marry at all. The result is that there is at least a 10- to 19-year period in which unmarried young men are having sex and at risk of making girls pregnant. These advocates believe that the most responsible program goal is to encourage abstinence but also to stress that sexually active young men should use contraception. . . .

A Combined Effort Is Necessary

All sectors, both public and private, should integrate a focus on males in current and future efforts to prevent pregnancy among teenage girls. Doing so will mean changing some prevention messages, adding some new messengers, and focusing on new and expanded audiences. If efforts to include boys and men in teen pregnancy are to be sustained, new leadership and new commitments of both volunteer time and funding from the public and private sectors will be required.

An important resource to involve in these efforts are national, state, and local youth-serving organizations that provide a variety of educational, recreational, and social services to boys and men, including the YMCAs, Boys and Girls Clubs of America, 100 Black Men of America, Inc., Big Brothers, Big Sisters of America, the National Urban League, and thousands of local youth development groups. Many involve older men from the community working directly with youth, particularly boys. The National Center on Fathers and Families at the University of Pennsylvania (215/573-5500) offers information on the growing number of community-based programs promoting responsible fatherhood. In addition, corporations, like Nike's P.L.A.Y. Foundation, and professional athletes—including basketball players David Robinson and A.C. Green and football player Darryl Green—are creating sports-based programming that appeals to boys and girls and offers them healthy opportunities. Such efforts to build a variety of skills among youth can help equip boys and young men with the motivation to avoid becoming fathers too soon.

As new male involvement initiatives grow and develop, the nation will move toward an understanding that teen pregnancy is the responsibility of both men and women, boys and girls. We must not be afraid to invest in rigorous evaluation of the best and most promising programs. And while more needs to be learned about effective approaches to helping boys and men play their part in avoiding teen pregnancy, existing programs have taught us important lessons. The challenge is to move from isolated innovation to sustained application so that male involvement becomes an integral part of all national, state, and local efforts to prevent teen pregnancy.

Periodical Bibliography

The following articles have been selected to supplement the diverse views presented in this chapter.

Sue Alford — "What's Wrong with Federal Abstinence-Only-Until-Marriage Requirements?" *Transitions*, March 2001.

Jacqueline Corcoran — "Preventing Adolescent Pregnancy: A Review of Programs and Practices," *Social Work*, January 2000.

Patricia Donovan — "Can Statutory Rape Laws Be Effective in Preventing Adolescent Pregnancy?" *Family Planning Perspectives*, January/February 1997.

Carol Ford — "Preventing Teen Pregnancy with Emergency Contraception: An Opportunity We Should Not Be Missing," *Archives of Pediatrics & Adolescent Medicine*, August 1998.

Donna Futterman — "Do Abstinence-Only Sex Education Programs Work?" *Family Practice News*, July 15, 2000.

Russell W. Gough — "The Hunt for the Sex-Education Truth," *World & I*, August 1997.

Alison Hadley — "How to Cut Teenage Pregnancies," *New Statesman*, July 3, 1998.

Debra W. Haffner — "What's Wrong with Abstinence-Only Sexuality Education Programs?" *SIECUS*, 1997.

Tamara Kreinin — "Keep Kids from Making Babies," *NEA Today*, November 1998.

Jodie Morse and Hillary Hylton — "Preaching Chastity in the Classroom," *Time*, October 18, 1999.

Sheron C. Patterson — "Churches Need to Teach Teens About Sex," *Dallas Morning News*, September 23, 2000.

Annys Shin — "OK, Boys and Girls—Don't Do It!" *National Journal*, October 25, 1997.

Gary Thomas — "True Love Waits," *Christianity Today*, March 1, 1999.

Paul V. Trad — "Assessing the Patterns That Prevent Teenage Pregnancy," *Adolescence*, Spring 1999.

For Further Discussion

Chapter 1

1. Kristin A. Moore and Barbara W. Sugland argue that although teenage pregnancy has declined since 1992, adolescent pregnancy is a serious problem in society. Janine Jackson claims that the problem of teenage pregnancy is exaggerated by the media. Whose argument do you find most convincing, and why?

2. Jasmine Miller argues that, given a chance, teenagers can make good parents. Lisa W. contends that teenage parenting is risky because teenage parents often suffer from a lack of education and poverty. With whose argument do you most agree? Explain your answer using examples from both texts.

Chapter 2

1. Linda Valdez and Ellen Goodman argue that enforcing statutory rape laws can reduce teenage pregnancy by deterring relationships between older men and teenage girls. Laura Duberstein Lindberg et al. contend that teenage parents are closer in age than some research suggests, so statutory rape laws may not be effective in reducing teenage pregnancy. Whose evidence do you find most persuasive and why?

2. Jacqueline L. Stock, Michelle A. Bell, Debra K. Boyer, and Frederick A. Connell argue that teenage girls who have suffered sexual abuse are more likely to engage in high-risk behaviors that may lead to pregnancy, such as unprotected sex and drug abuse, than girls who have not been abused. Do you find their argument persuasive? Why, or why not? What factors other than sexual abuse contribute to high-risk behavior and teenage pregnancy?

3. Jo Ann Wentzel contends that inaccurate sex information contributes to teenage pregnancy. Do you agree with her contention? Using information in this book, assess the accuracy of your own knowledge of sex and sexuality.

Chapter 3

1. Elisabeth Pruden relates her personal experience as a pregnant teenager who opted for abortion and maintains that although the decision was difficult, she does not regret the choice she made. Liz Kleemeier, as the product of a teenage pregnancy who was adopted at birth, contends that women should not have

the option of aborting babies who could otherwise be adopted by loving families. Whose personal story do you find the most persuasive, and why?

2. Rebecca Lanning describes the story of Amy, a teenage mother who gave her baby up for adoption. Amy contends that the family she chose to adopt her son could offer him more financial and familial stability than she could. Based on evidence in the text, do you think that Amy made a wise decision? Why or why not?

3. Katha Pollitt maintains that only 3 percent of white girls and 1 percent of black girls choose adoption as a solution for an unplanned teenage pregnancy. Why do you think so few girls choose adoption? Do you think more girls should be encouraged to carry their babies to term and give them up for adoption? Why, or why not?

Chapter 4

1. According to the Planned Parenthood Federation of America, traditional sex education that teaches students the biology of sex and how to protect themselves from pregnancy and sexually transmitted diseases can reduce teenage pregnancy. Lakita Garth maintains that abstinence-only education, which teaches students to refrain from sex until marriage, is the best way to reduce teenage pregnancy. Whose argument do you find the most convincing, and why? How do you think sex education should be taught in schools?

2. Lakita Garth argues that abstinence education should not only teach students to abstain from sex until marriage, but also teach them the valuable lessons of "self-control, self-discipline, and the delay of self-gratification." How do you think the pursuit of self-control, self-discipline, and delay of self-gratification relates to sexuality? Do you agree with her argument? Why, or why not?

3. Isabel V. Sawhill maintains that provisions of the 1996 welfare reform bill may help reduce incidents of teenage pregnancy by making it more difficult for teenage parents to obtain and rely on welfare benefits. Kathleen Sylvester contends that the current welfare system does not reduce teenage pregnancy because the high number of welfare recipients in poverty-stricken neighborhoods makes welfare dependency seem like an acceptable life path to impressionable teenage girls. Do you think that the welfare system contributes to teenage pregnancy? How do you

think young girls could escape a family history of welfare dependency? Explain your answer.

4. Kristin A. Moore et al. argue that sex education programs often neglect to educate teenage boys in their role in teenage pregnancy prevention. Do you think that adolescent boys are taught enough about preventing pregnancy? How would you formulate a sex education curriculum that targeted both boys and girls?

Organizations to Contact

The editors have compiled the following list of organizations concerned with the issues debated in this book. The descriptions are derived from materials provided by the organizations. All have publications or information available for interested readers. The list was compiled on the date of publication of the present volume; names, addresses, phone and fax numbers, and e-mail and Internet addresses may change. Be aware that many organizations take several weeks or longer to respond to inquiries, so allow as much time as possible.

Advocates for Youth
1025 Vermont Ave. NW, Suite 200, Washington, DC 20005
(202) 347-5700 • fax: (202) 347-2263
e-mail: Info@advocatesforyouth.org
website: www.advocatesforyouth.org

Formerly the Center for Population Options, Advocates for Youth is the only national organization focusing solely on pregnancy and HIV prevention among young people. It provides information, education, and advocacy to youth-serving agencies and professionals, policy makers, and the media. Among the organization's numerous publications are the brochures "Advice from Teens on Buying Condoms" and "Spread the Word—Not the Virus" and the pamphlet *How to Prevent Date Rape: Teen Tips*.

The Alan Guttmacher Institute
120 Wall St., New York, NY 10005
(212) 248-1111 • fax: (212) 248-1951
e-mail: info@agi-usa.org • website: www.agi-usa.org

The institute works to protect and expand the reproductive choices of all women and men. It strives to ensure people's access to the information and services they need to exercise their rights and responsibilities concerning sexual activity, reproduction, and family planning. Among the institute's publications are the books *Teenage Pregnancy in Industrialized Countries* and *Today's Adolescents, Tomorrow's Parents: A Portrait of the Americas* and the report "Sex and America's Teenagers."

Child Trends, Inc. (CT)
4301 Connecticut Ave. NW, Suite 100, Washington, DC 20008
(202) 362-5580 • fax: (202) 362-5533
website: www.childtrends.org

CT works to provide accurate statistical and research information regarding children and their families in the United States and to educate the American public on the ways existing social trends—such as the increasing rate of teenage pregnancy—affect children. In addition to the newsletter *Facts at a Glance*, which presents the latest data on teen pregnancy rates for every state, CT also publishes the papers "Next Steps and Best Bets: Approaches to Preventing Adolescent Childbearing" and "Welfare and Adolescent Sex: The Effects of Family History, Benefit Levels, and Community Context."

Concerned Women for America (CWA)
1015 15th St. NW, Suite 1100, Washington, DC 20005
(202) 488-7000 • fax: (202) 488-0806
website: www.cwfa.org

CWA's purpose is to preserve, protect, and promote traditional Judeo-Christian values through education, legislative action, and other activities. It is concerned with creating an environment that is conducive to building strong families and raising healthy children. CWA publishes the monthly *Family Voice*, which periodically addresses issues such as abortion and promoting sexual abstinence in schools.

Family Research Council
801 G St. NW, Washington, DC 20001
(202) 393-2100 • fax: (202) 393-2134
website: www.frc.org

The council seeks to promote and protect the interests of the traditional family. It focuses on issues such as parental autonomy and responsibility, community support for single parents, and adolescent pregnancy. Among the council's numerous publications are the papers "Revolt of the Virgins," "Abstinence: The New Sexual Revolution," and "Abstinence Programs Show Promise in Reducing Sexual Activity and Pregnancy Among Teens."

Family Resource Coalition (FRC)
200 S. Michigan Ave., 16th Fl., Chicago, IL 60604
(312) 341-0900 • fax: (312) 341-9361

The FRC is a national consulting and advocacy organization that seeks to strengthen and empower families and communities so they can foster the optimal development of children, teenagers, and adult family members. The FRC publishes the bimonthly newsletter *Connection*, the report "Family Involvement in Adolescent Pregnancy and Parenting Programs," and the fact sheet "Family Support Programs and Teen Parents."

Focus on the Family
8605 Explorer Dr., Colorado Springs, CO 80920
(719) 531-5181 • fax: (719) 531-3424
website: www.family.org

Focus on the Family is a Christian organization dedicated to preserving and strengthening the traditional family. It believes that the breakdown of the traditional family is in part linked to increases in teen pregnancy, and so it conducts research on the ethics of condom use and the effectiveness of safe-sex education programs in schools. The organization publishes the video *Sex, Lies, and the Truth*, which discusses the issue of teen sexuality and abstinence, as well as *Brio*, a monthly magazine for teenage girls.

Girls, Inc.
30 E. 33rd St., New York, NY 10016-5394
(212) 689-3700 • fax: (212) 683-1253

Girls, Inc. is an organization for girls aged six to eighteen that works to create an environment in which girls can learn and grow to their full potential. It conducts daily programs in career and life planning, health and sexuality, and leadership and communication. Girls, Inc. publishes the newsletter *Girls Ink* six times a year, which provides information of interest to young girls and women, including information on teen pregnancy.

The Heritage Foundation
214 Massachusetts Ave. NE, Washington, DC 20002
(202) 546-4400 • fax: (202) 546-0904
website: www.nhf.org

The Heritage Foundation is a public policy research institute that supports the ideas of limited government and the free-market system. It promotes the view that the welfare system has contributed to the problems of illegitimacy and teenage pregnancy. Among the foundation's numerous publications is its Backgrounder series, which includes "Liberal Welfare Programs: What the Data Show on Programs for Teenage Mothers"; the paper "Rising Illegitimacy: America's Social Catastrophe"; and the bulletin "How Congress Can Protect the Rights of Parents to Raise Their Children."

The Manhattan Institute
52 Vanderbilt Ave., New York, NY 10017
(212) 599-7000 • fax: (212) 599-3494
e-mail: info@manhattan-institute.org
website: www.manhattan-institute.org

The institute is a nonpartisan research organization that seeks to educate scholars, government officials, and the public on the economy and how government programs affect it. It publishes the quarterly magazine *City Journal* and the article "The Teen Mommy Track."

National Campaign to Prevent Teen Pregnancy
1776 Massachusetts Ave. NW, Suite 200, Washington, DC 20036
(202) 478-8500
website: www.teenpregnancy.org

The goal of the National Campaign to Prevent Teen Pregnancy is to prevent teen pregnancy by supporting values and stimulating actions that are consistent with a pregnancy-free adolescence. The organization publishes the report "Whatever Happened to Childhood? The Problem of Teen Pregnancy in the United States."

National Organization of Adolescent Pregnancy, Parenting, and Prevention (NOAPPP)
1319 F St. NW, Suite 401, Washington, DC 20004
(202) 783-5770 • fax: (202) 783-5775
e-mail: noapp@aol.com

NOAPPP promotes comprehensive and coordinated services designed for the prevention and resolution of problems associated with adolescent pregnancy and parenthood. It supports families in setting standards that encourage the healthy development of children through loving, stable relationships. NOAPPP publishes the quarterly *NOAPPP Network Newsletter* and various fact sheets on teen pregnancy.

Planned Parenthood Federation of America (PPFA)
810 Seventh Ave., New York, NY 10019
(212) 541-7800 • fax: (212) 245-1845
website: www.plannedparenthood.org

PPFA is a national organization that supports people's right to make their own reproductive decisions without governmental interference. In 1989, it developed First Things First, a nationwide adolescent pregnancy prevention program. This program promotes the view that every child has the right to secure an education, attain physical and emotional maturity, and establish life goals before assuming the responsibilities of parenthood. Among PPFA's numerous publications are the booklets *Teen Sex?*, *Facts About Birth Control*, and *How to Talk with Your Teen About the Facts of Life*.

Progressive Policy Institute (PPI)
600 Pennsylvania Ave. SE, Suite 400, Washington, DC 20003
(202) 546-0007
website: www.dlcppi.org

The PPI is a public policy research organization that strives to develop alternatives to the traditional debate between the left and the right. It advocates social policies designed to liberate the poor from poverty and dependence. The institute publishes *Reducing Teenage Pregnancy: A Handbook for Action* and the reports "Second-Chance Homes: Breaking the Cycle of Teen Pregnancy" and "Preventable Calamity: Rolling Back Teen Pregnancy."

Religious Coalition for Reproductive Choice
1025 Vermont Ave. NW, Suite 1130, Washington, DC 20005
(202) 628-7700 • fax: (202) 628-7716
e-mail: info@rcrc.org • website: www.rcrc.org

The coalition works to inform the media and the public that many mainstream religions support reproductive options, including abortion, and oppose antiabortion violence. It works to mobilize pro-choice religious people to counsel families facing unintended pregnancies. The coalition publishes "The Role of Religious Congregations in Fostering Adolescent Sexual Health," "Abortion: Finding Your Own Truth," and "Considering Abortion? Clarify What You Believe."

The Robin Hood Foundation
111 Broadway, 19th Fl., New York, NY 10006
(212) 227-6601 • fax: (212) 227-6698
website: www.robinhood.org

The Robin Hood Foundation makes grants to early childhood, youth, and family-centered programs located in the five boroughs of New York City. It publishes the report "Kids Having Kids: A Robin Hood Foundation Special Report on the Costs of Adolescent Childbearing."

Sexuality Information and Education Council of the United States (SIECUS)
130 W. 42nd St., Suite 350, New York, NY 10036-7802
(212) 819-9770 • fax: (212) 819-9776
e-mail: SIECUS@siecus.org • website: www.siecus.org

SIECUS develops, collects, and disseminates information on human sexuality. It promotes comprehensive education about sexuality and advocates the right of individuals to make responsible sexual choices. In addition to providing guidelines for sexuality education for kindergarten through twelfth grades, SIECUS publishes the reports "Facing Facts: Sexual Health for America's Adolescents" and "Teens Talk About Sex: Adolescent Sexuality in the 90s" and the fact sheet "Adolescents and Abstinence."

Teen STAR Program
Natural Family Planning Center of Washington, D.C.
8514 Bradmoor Dr., Bethesda, MD 20817-3810
(301) 897-9323 • fax: (301) 571-5267
e-mail: hklaus@dgsys.com • website: www2.dgsys.com

Teen STAR (Sexuality Teaching in the context of Adult Responsibility) is geared for early, middle, and late adolescence. Classes are designed to foster understanding of the body and its fertility pattern and to explore the emotional, cognitive, social, and spiritual aspects of human sexuality. Teen STAR publishes a bimonthly newsletter and the paper "Sexual Behavior of Youth: How to Influence It."

Bibliography of Books

Shirley Arthur — *Surviving Teen Pregnancy: Your Choices, Dreams, and Decisions*. Minneapolis, MN: Econo-clad, 1999.

Linda Barr, Catherine Monserrat, and Toni Berg — *Working with Pregnant and Parenting Teens: A Guide for Use with Teenage Pregnancy*. Albuquerque, NM: New Futures, 1996.

Edmund F. Benson and Susan Benson — *Teen Pregnancy*. Miami, FL: ARISE Foundation, 1997.

Kay Beyer — *Coping with Teen Parenting*. New York: Rosen, 1999.

Janet Bode, Stanley Mack, and Ida Marx Blue Spruce — *Kids Still Having Kids: Talking About Teen Pregnancy*. Danbury, CT: Franklin Watts, 1999.

Ginny Brinkley — *Baby and Me: A Pregnancy Workbook for Young Women*. New York: Pink Inc! 1997.

Cynthia Cass — *Success After Teen Pregnancy: Against All Odds*. Kearney, NE: Morris, 1998.

Janet Ollila Colberg and Joel Nakamura — *Red Light Green Light: Preventing Teen Pregnancy*. Helena, MT: Summer Kitchen, 1997.

Julie K. Endersbe — *Teen Fathers: Getting Involved*. Santa Rosa, CA: Lifematters, 2000.

Christine Flanigan — *What's Behind the Good News: The Decline in Teen Pregnancy During the 1990s*. Washington, DC: National Campaign to Prevent Teen Pregnancy, 2001.

Maggie Gallagher, David Blankenhorn, and Milton Avery — *Age of Unwed Mothers: Is Teen Pregnancy the Problem?* New York: Institute for American Values, 1999.

Ted Gottfried — *Teen Fathers Today*. Breckenridge, CO: Twenty First Century, 2001.

Jane Hammerslough — *Everything You Need to Know About Teen Motherhood*. New York: Rosen, 2001.

John Hutchins — *Next Best Thing: Helping Sexually Active Teens Avoid Pregnancy*. Washington, DC: National Campaign to Prevent Teen Pregnancy, 2000.

Raymond Jamiolkowski — *A Baby Doesn't Make the Man: Alternative Sources of Power and Manhood for Young Men*. New York: Rosen, 1997.

Douglas Kirby	*No Easy Answers: Research Findings on Programs to Reduce Teen Pregnancies.* Washington, DC: National Campaign to Prevent Teen Pregnancy, 1997.
Anna Kreiner and Janice Goodall	*In Control: Learning to Say No to Sexual Pressure.* New York: Rosen, 1999.
Susan Kuklin	*What Do I Do Now? Talking About Teen Pregnancy.* Lincoln, NE: Writers Club/iUniverse.com, 2001.
Evelyn Lerman and Jami Moffett	*Teen Moms: The Pain and the Promise.* Buena Park, CA: Morning Glory, 1997.
Rebecca A. Maynard	*Kids Having Kids: Economic Costs and Social Consequences of Teen Pregnancy.* Washington, DC: Urban Institute, 1996.
Luther B. McIntyre	*Help for Hurting Parents: Dealing with the Pain of Teen Pregnancy.* San Francisco, CA: Good Life, 1998.
Barbara Miller	*Teen Pregnancy and Poverty: The Economic Realities.* New York: Rosen, 1997.
Barbara A. Moe	*A Question of Timing: Successful Men Talk About Having Children.* New York: Rosen, 1997.
National Campaign to Prevent Teen Pregnancy	*What About the Teens? Research on What Teens Say About Teen Pregnancy: A Focus Group Study.* Washington, DC: National Campaign to Prevent Teen Pregnancy, 1999.
Sudie Pollock, Jeanne Warren, ed., and David Warren	*Will the Dollars Stretch? Teen Parents Living on Their Own: Virtual Reality Through Stories and Checkwriting Practice.* Buena Park, CA: Morning Glory, 1997.
Isabel V. Sawhill and John Hutchins	*Ready Resources: Investing Welfare Funds in Teen Pregnancy Prevention.* Washington, DC: National Campaign to Prevent Teen Pregnancy, 2000.
Linda I. Shands	*What Now? Help for Pregnant Teens.* Westmont, IL: InterVarsity, 1999.
Christopher Shays, ed.	*Preventing Teen Pregnancy: Coordinating Community Efforts.* Collingdale, PA: Diane, 1999.
P.L. Sunderland and Joan E. O'Brien	*Why I Waited: Successful Women Talk About Their Pregnancy Choices.* New York: Rosen, 1997.
Margi Trapani	*Listen Up! Teenage Mothers Speak Out.* New York: Rosen, 1997.
James Wong and David Checkland, eds.	*Teen Pregnancy and Parenting: Social and Ethical Issues.* Ontario, Canada: University of Toronto Press, 2000.

Index

abortion
  should be an option for pregnant
    teenagers, 86–92
  con, 93–97
  teenage, decline in, 85
abstinence
  as a lifestyle, 114
  promotion of
    in male involvement programs,
      174
    in sexual education programs,
      136
abstinence education
  can reduce teenage pregnancy,
    113–22
  con, 123–33
  does not delay sexual activity,
    129
  evaluation of, is lacking, 23
  welfare reform and, 125–27, 149
Adolescent Family Life Act of
  1981 (AFLA), 124, 126–27
adoption
  is an option for pregnant
    teenagers, 98–105
  con, 106–109
  problems with, 108
African Americans
  fathers, decline in economic
    status of, 158
  males, gap between first
    intercourse and marriage
    among, 165
  teenage birth rates among, 21
age differences
  in relationships, cultural
    attitudes on, 48
Alan Guttmacher Institute, 12,
  137
  on welfare reform, 14–15
alcohol
  risk of, to babies, 45
  use of, association with mother-
    father age gap, 59
Alstad, Diana, 85
American Academy of Pediatrics,
  13
American Journal of Public Health,
  50

Anderson, Elijah, 74
Arizona Department of Health
  Services, 50
Atlanta Journal and Constitution
  (newspaper), 29

behavior problems
  mother-father age gaps and, 58
  as risk factor for teenage
    pregnancy, 23
Bell, Michelle A., 63
Best Friends program, 117
birth rates, teenage, 17, 115
  recent trends in, 20–21
  volatility of, 22
births
  low birth weight
    costs of, 156
    teenagers' risks for, 135
  out-of-wedlock, 115, 147–48
bisexual youths
  pregnancy among, 141
Boyer, Debra K., 63
Burnett, Gilbert H., 120, 121

California Department of Health
  Services, 52
Carrera, Michael A., 14
Castle, Michael N., 75
Chew, Kenneth S.Y., 50, 55
Chicago Sun-Times (newspaper), 28
childbearing, teenage
  adverse consequences of, 12,
    121, 135
  most youth avoid, 30
  arguments against, 81–82
  factors placing youth at risk of,
    22–23
  is a symptom, not cause of
    problems, 73
  most occurs outside of marriage,
    148
  reasons for, 158–60
  social costs of, 12, 17, 44, 135,
    156–57
children, of teenage mothers
  risk of poor outcomes to, 20, 45,
    135, 155, 156
Choosing the Best (curriculum),

130–31
Clark, Susan, 35
Cleveland Plain Dealer (newspaper), 28, 29, 31, 32
Clinton, Bill, 29, 31, 32, 107
Clinton, Hillary Rodham, 72
Connell, Frederick A., 63
contraceptives
    AIDS education increases use of, 134
    need for information on, 137
    public funding for, 139–41
    teens need easy access to, 138–39
    teen use of, 125
        among males, 165
Coontz, Stephanie, 29
Cooper, Richard T., 71
Curren, Eric, 119

Dechman, Margaret, 36
Detroit News (newspaper), 28

education
    teenage childbearing limits opportunities for, 12–13, 43
        con, 36
Elton, Catherine, 48

Fagan, Patrick F., 13, 18
FAIR (Fairness and Accuracy in Reporting), 27
families
    problems in, as risk factor for teenage birth, 22
    single-parent
        association with child poverty and, 145–46
        increase in, 17
        welfare system normalizes, 157
Felix, Shannon, 34–35, 36–37, 38–41
Fetal Alcohol Syndrome, 45
Flinn, Susan K., 69
Forrest, J.D., 55

Garth, Lakita, 113
Geronimus, Arline T., 74
Goodman, Ellen, 49

Haffner, Debra W., 112, 140
Harris, Damien, 118–19
Hispanics

males, gap between first intercourse and marriage among, 165
    teenage birth rates among, 21
Hotz, Joseph, 71, 74

income
    association with mother-father age gap, 58–59
In These Times (Males), 31

Jackson, Janine, 27

Kids Count, 13
Kleemeier, Liz, 93
Klein, Joe, 30
Korenman, Sanders, 74
Krauthammer, Charles, 31
Ku, Leighton, 54

Landry, D.S., 55
Lanning, Rebecca, 98
lesbian youths
    pregnancy among, 141
Lindberg, Laura Duberstein, 54, 169
Lisa W., 42
Lopez, Aurora, 73–74
Los Compadres, 172
Luker, Kristin, 108

Mahler, K., 103
male involvement programs
    structuring of, 170–71
    types of, 168–70
males
    gap between first intercourse and marriage among, 165
    involvement programs for, can reduce teenage pregnancy, 164–75
    media images of, 172–73
    older
        contribute to teenage pregnancy, 31, 49–53, 141
            con, 54–62
        disincentives for, to father child with minor, 61–62
    teenage
        developmental stages of, 167–68
        have role in pregnancy

prevention, 141–42, 169
need for mentors/role models
  for, 171
vs. women, age differences in
  relationships, 48
Males, Mike, 31, 50, 55
marriage
  delays in, and sexual activity,
    151, 162–63, 165, 174
  effects of sexual revolution on,
    17
Marsiglio, William, 166
Martinez, Gladys, 54
Maternal and Child Health Block
  Grant program, 125
Mayers, Rodney, 36, 40
McIlhaney, Joe, 112, 117
McKinnon, Margaret, 37
media
  exaggerates problem of teenage
    pregnancy, 27–32
  male images in, 172–73
  presents distorted messages
    about sex, 128
Miller, Jasmine, 33
Milwaukee Sentinel (newspaper), 30
Mincy, Ronald, 158
Moore, Kristin A., 19, 23, 77
Murray, Charles, 28, 32

National Abortion and
  Reproductive Rights Action
  League, 95, 123
National Campaign to Prevent
  Teen Pregnancy, 12, 52, 72, 129,
  131–32, 165
National Council for Adoption,
  108
National Maternal and Infant
  Health Survey, 58
National Right to Life
  Committee, 95
National Survey of Adolescent
  Men, 166
National Survey of Families and
  Households, 158
National Survey of Family
  Growth, 137
National Teens for Life, 96
neighborhood opportunity
  centers, 161–62
New York Times (newspaper), 31

Oberman, Michelle, 53
Ooms, Theodora, 164
out-of-wedlock births, 115
  loss of stigma attached to,
    147–48

Parenting Today's Teen (online
  publication), 78
Pernas, Marta, 169
Personal Responsibility and Work
  Opportunity Reconciliation Act,
  14
physical abuse
  link with teenage pregnancy, 70,
    141
Planned Parenthood Federation of
  America, 95, 96, 134
Pollitt, Katha, 106
poverty
  child, association with single-
    parent families, 145–46
  link with teenage childbearing,
    13–14, 22, 71–77
  is questionable, 29
  as risk factor for teenage birth,
    22
  teens in, need for publicly funded
    family planning for, 139–42
pregnancy
  myths about, 79–81
  teenage
    abstinence-only sex education
      can reduce, 113–22
    con, 123–33
    is a serious problem, 19–26
    lack of accurate sex information
      contributes to, 78–82
    among lesbians/bisexuals, 141
    may mask sexual abuse, 69
    media exaggerates problem of,
      27–32
    older men contribute to, 49–53
    as a political issue, 76–77
    poor life circumstances
      contribute to, 71–77
    prevention of, 44–45
      male involvement programs
        for, 164–75
      media's role in, 138
      need for public funding for,
        139–42
    welfare reform and, 149

rates for, 135
  are declining, 144–45
  in Canada, 35
  in U.S. vs. Europe, 107–108
  sexual abuse contributes to, 31,
    63–70, 141
  social costs of, 120–21
  welfare benefits do not reduce,
    143–53
  welfare reform may reduce,
    143–53
  unintended, in U.S., 128
premature births
  teenagers' risks for, 44–45, 135
Pruden, Elisabeth, 86

rape
  teen pregnancies resulting from,
    31
  of underage females, 51
risk factors
  for teenage childbearing, 22–23
Rites of Passage Collective, 172
Robinson, Khadija, 73–74
Rollin, Betty, 31

Sawhill, Isabel V., 143
Scales, Peter C., 30
second-chance homes, 160–61
sex education
  abstinence-only
    can reduce teenage pregnancy,
      113–22
    evaluation of, is lacking, 23
  availability of, 151
  does not encourage sexual
    activity, 132
  lack of, contributes to teenage
    pregnancy, 78–82
  public support for, 132–33, 136
  traditional, can reduce teenage
    pregnancy, 24
Sex Respect (curriculum), 130
sexual abuse
  contributes to teenage
    pregnancy, 31, 63–70, 141
sexual activity
  abstinence education does not
    delay, 129
  comprehensive sexuality
    education does not encourage,
    132

delay of marriage and, 151,
    162–63, 165, 174
  male, key facts about, 165–66
  peer pressure and, 150–51
sexually transmitted diseases
  (STDs)
  abstinence education does not
    address, 124
  misinformation about, 128
  prevalence of, 115, 125, 157
sexual revolution
  casualties of, 119–20
  views on sexuality and marriage
    affected by, 17
Shriver, Eunice Kennedy, 115
Smith, Susan, 95
Sonenstein, Freya L., 54, 169
Starr, Oliver, Jr., 52
statutory rape laws, 50, 56
  enforcement of, 51–52, 55
    is unlikely to affect teen
      childbearing, 61
  welfare reform and, 149
Stock, Jacqueline L., 63
St. Thomas Plain Talk Project, 172
Sugland, Barbara W., 19, 23
surveys
  on attitudes toward sexual
    activity, 151–52, 166
  on parents providing sex
    education, 127
  on sexual abuse of teens, 67–68
  on teenage births fathered by
    older men, 50, 52, 56–57
    link with race and income, 58
  on wanted births to teenage
    mothers, 158
Sylvester, Kathleen, 154

Teachers for Life Association, 85
Teenage Pregnancy Prevention
  Act of 1995 (California), 56
teenagers
  adult views on sexuality of, 37
  can make good parents, 33–41
    con, 42–45
  lesbian/bisexual, pregnancy
    among, 141
  male, developmental stages of,
    167–68
  motivating factors to avoid
    pregnancy, 25–26

Teen Aid (curriculum), 131
Time (magazine), 32
Turcios, Miriam, 77

Urban Institute, 30, 48

Valdez, Linda, 49
Villarosa, Linda, 48

Wall Street Journal (newspaper), 28, 32
Washington Alliance Concerned with School Age Parents, 50
Washington Post (newspaper), 29
Washington State Survey of Adolescent Health Behaviors, 65
welfare
 alternatives to, 160–62
 benefits do not reduce teenage pregnancy, 30, 154–63
 utilization of, by teen mothers, 17–18

Welfare Reform Act of 1996, 14, 112, 143
 abstinence education and, 125–27
 may reduce teenage pregnancy, 143–53
 measures to reduce teen births in, are punitive, 14–15
 requirements of, 148–50
 see also Personal Responsibility and Work Opportunity Reconciliation Act
Wentzel, Jo Ann, 78
Westheimer, Ruth, 116
Wetstein, Cheryl, 120
Williams, Sean, 169
Wilson, Pete, 51–52, 72
Wilson, William Julius, 60
Wong, Donna, 44
World Health Organization, 132

Zabin, Laurie Schwab, 158